Postherpetic Neuralgia Explained

Shingles virus

Postherpetic neuralgia symptoms, postherpetic neuralgia treatment, post-shingles pain, herpetic neuralgia, all covered

By Milica Jovanovic

Published by Cleal Publishing

Copyright ©2017 Cleal Publishing

ISBN (978-0-9955610-4-5)

Copyright

All rights reserved. No part of this book may be reproduced or transferred in any form or by any means, graphic, electronic, or mechanical, including photocopying, recording, taping, or by any information storage retrieval system, without the written permission of the publisher.

Disclaimer

While the author and publisher have made all available efforts to ensure the information contained in this book was correct as of press time, neither the author nor publisher assumes and hereby disclaims any liability to any party for damages, disruption, or loss caused by the use and application, directly or indirectly, of any information presented including any errors. This book is not meant to substitute for medical advice from a qualified healthcare professional. The reader should regularly consult with a healthcare professional in matters relating to his/her health, particularly with respect to any of the symptoms discussed that may require professional treatment. The accuracy and completeness of information provided herein and opinions stated herein are not guaranteed or warranted to produce any particular results, and the advice and strategies contained herein may not be suitable for every individual.

Introduction

Herpetic pain after viral herpes zoster infection is a burden that many people struggle with, and yet the treatment that would completely relieve pain is only a partial solution. The question is how to handle such pain, which isn't caused by visible injury and, after the inflammation is long gone, the pain persists. There is some misinformation about a lot of things concerning shingles, the way it is acquired, what should be done, and what shouldn't be done. Generally, the severest problem is to manage the pain, which is a complication of herpes zoster infection that can affect the quality of living, working, and sleeping. To clarify, here are the facts about the virus, its influence on the body, and its characteristics, as well as what can be done to treat and prevent further complications and prolonged pain.

The pain and nerve damage may be successfully prevented and treated with the right type of treatment for each individual who is immunocompromised and doesn't seem to have many options for the treatment of such pain. The new medications are fighting against this false perception of pain of neuropathic pain and neuralgia, which happen in herpes zoster and have a great impact on everyday life. This false perception comes from damaged nerves and it is the brain that induces such terrible pain. The question is: How much pain is bearable for each person and do we actually need to suffer and endure it? Do we have to feel so limited and restricted from doing anything because the pain is entrapping us? No. Is there a solution to not measure any daily activity with how painful it could be? Yes. The goal can be achieved and the pain, if not eliminated, can be decreased and the quality of life much improved.

Chapter 1

Postherpetic neuralgia is a common problem and is more and more often found after infection with the herpes zoster virus. The virus functions in many ways that are yet to be discovered and explained by humans. They are small, smaller than bacteria and, more often than not, they reactivate inside the living cells of an organism, causing specific changes, mutations, damage to specific structures, etc. Some of the virus remains hidden in the body. The treatment needs to focus entirely on immunity and ways to repress the viral effects on the genome and structures and also on the function of the cells and organs.

This virus that induces herpes zoster is neurotropic, which means that it has a certain affinity for nerve cells, and it binds and affects them. This is how the neuralgia develops—when the nerves become damaged and begin to malfunction. This happens most often when immunity is lower and doesn't act against the virus. The elder population is the group of people most vulnerable to herpes zoster and postherpetic neuralgia. They may have these symptoms for as long as a year.

It is important to take a look at the structure and characteristics of this virus, and possible ways how it can be defeated, in order to find a solution for pain and other complications of herpes zoster.

Etiology

Herpes zoster (shingles) virus and varicella

Herpes zoster virus belongs to a family of viruses, *Herpesviridae*, which is divided into classes A, B, and C. Herpesviridae share one characteristic, latency of appearance and a constant presence in the body, and yet they only induce symptoms and illness in certain circumstances, which is how they got their name (Greek *herpein*, to hide). They appear to be hidden in the body, not inducing any symptoms, unless the body is in a certain state.

Among Herpesviridae, the most common in our population are herpes simplex virus (types 1 and 2), which induces herpes on the lips (type 1) or genitals (type 2); cytomegalovirus (CMV), which induces mononucleosis syndrome (sore throat, rash, enlargement of the liver and spleen); Epstein-Barr virus (EBV), which also induces mononucleosis syndrome but in additions is responsible for some forms of cancer in the throat and lymphoma; and, of course, the varicella zoster virus (VZV), which induces varicella in children and adults and herpes zoster in adults.

Table 1 Table of Herpes viruses

α Herpseviridae	Herpes simplex type 1
	Herpes simplex type 2
	Varicella zoster virus
ß Herpesviridae	Cytomegalovirus (CMV)
ɣ Herpesviridae	Epstein-Barr (EBV)

Varicella is better known as the chicken pox. It is a common, highly contagious, but benign disease that affects mostly children, but sometimes adults as well. The virus is spread through the air, i.e., inhaling the particles when someone coughs, sneezes, speaks loudly, etc. It presents with high fever, malaise, a rash that starts at the abdomen by forming red spots, which quickly turn into itchy blisters that fill with pus, but then turn into crusts. This rash doesn't appear all at once, but rather in waves, which is why there are skin rashes of different stadia that are present and become visible at the same time. The rash spreads centripetally, which means from the abdomen to the head and hairy part of the head and outward to the extremities. The child needs to be isolated while it has the rash and it is actually contagious for others 1-2 days before the symptoms occur. The illness lasts usually approximately seven days, and complete resolution of symptoms may take seven more days. In smaller children, varicella can be barely noticeable, and is easily treated with medications for fever and muscle and joint pain, but only with paracetamol, because aspirin may lead to Reyes syndrome, an especially dangerous occurrence in children.

In young adults, varicella can be complicated with pneumonia, inflammation of the lung lobes, which then requires specific treatment. Also, pregnant women, the elderly, and adults with low immunity are more sensitive and prone to complications, so they should visit a doctor's office for assessment. Varicella is the first manifestation if the first contact of the body with the virus. After the primoinfection, the virus is suppressed by the immunological system, and banished into the ganglions, since they are, as previously mentioned, neurotropic viruses. They remain hidden in the ganglions; they are not destroyed, but they do not interfere with normal body functioning.

Herpes zoster or shingles

After the resolution of chickenpox, the virus doesn't leave the body, but rather stays hidden in the ganglions of the nerves, from where it can induce one more attack when the immunity drops. However, the second illness is different, because once the virus has been beaten, the immunological response grows strong to prevent another infection from the same cause or to decrease the impact of the virus if it attacks again. In the elderly and people with lowered immunity, varicella zoster virus will induce another similar illness, which is now associated with inflammation to the nerve, which we call herpes zoster or shingles. The virus will travel through the pathway of a nerve to the skin and cause a localized infection, limited to one part of the body, on one side.

Epidemiology

Varicella appears today as a common disease which, in many cases, stays unreported for its benign course. It is important to evaluate the rate of people who are not immunized against varicella and are adults or pregnant women. This is under 5% in the USA, around 16% in Saudi Arabia, and up to 50% in Sri Lanka. This means that, in the US, as many as 95% of the people have had a contact with varicella zoster and gained immunity against it but, in contrast to that, people in Sri Lanka are vulnerable to new infections of herpes zoster because this virus and illness are not as present in their population. Varicella is not widespread in countries that have a tropical climate. The incidence of herpes zoster is lower because not everyone who had chicken pox in childhood will have a shingles infection.

Elderly people are more prone to develop singles, and half of the people who are 85 years old have had at least one episode of shingles in their lifetime. Those older than 50 years have a bigger chance of developing shingles, since immunity begins to slowly drop at that age. (1) Viruses activate a special type of immunity, cell immunity, rather than antibodies, and cell immunity declines with age and the presence of some other illnesses and conditions. The immunological response in the cells is triggered when the virus enters the cells. Between 20% and 30% of all people who have had chickenpox will develop shingles at least once in their lifetime. If we take a look at reports of the incidence before the age of 50 years and compare them to today's statistics, there would be a significant increase in incidence today, which is yet to be explained. (2) This may be explained in positive reasons because people's lifespan has increased. Also, there are many illnesses that deprive people of immunity, and that is the key factor in developing herpes zoster.

Many people have only one occurrence of shingles, while other may have two or three or more episodes of shingles. The accurate data is impossible to gather. Not all of the ill people seek medical help and get noted in the statistical data, and most of the mild infections pass spontaneously with mild symptomatic treatment. However, sometimes hospitalization is required, especially when the doctors aren't exactly sure of the diagnosis in the first phase or when complications develop in the second phase. The rate of hospitalization is between 1% and 4%, which speaks about the incidence of complications.

People who have received the varicella vaccine for any reason, have already activated their immunological response, but with subtle symptoms. The vaccine prevents complications at the first contact with the virus, which is a benefit. Another good outcome of vaccination is that there is a smaller chance of developing herpes zoster if a child is vaccinated than if it becomes ill with varicella at a young age. It may help to know that there is a smaller chance of developing shingles in children and in people who have become ill from some immunocompromising condition.

Risk factors

There are some risk factors that should be considered as possible triggers for shingles:

- People who have had chickenpox or who were vaccinated against VZV already have viral particles in the organism and the outcome entirely depends on the immunological status;
- People more than 50 years old;
- People with any type of cancer have lower immunity in general;
- People who are HIV-positive or have AIDS, because in these illnesses cell immunity gets lower and lower through the years;
- People who have had bone marrow or any other transplantation;
- People who take prescribed medications to lower their immunity in autoimmune diseases and other diseases and transplantation, where the immunological system doesn't work properly and "attacks" their own cells—these medications are referred to as immunosuppressives, and among them, there are corticosteroids, cytostatics, 5-ASA and others;

- People who have received chemotherapy or radiation treatment;
- People with diabetes are prone to any type of infection including shingles;
- People who suffer from stress or a traumatic experience;
- People who have had severe injuries;
- A child of a pregnant woman who has had varicella in pregnancy is at risk to develop shingles during the first two years of its life, even though it is generally rare for children to develop shingles.

The immunological system prevents another infection from arising and, after chickenpox, most of the body is cleared of the virus and it becomes suppressed to only one or a couple of locations, which become the predisposing locations for shingles. The skin lesions appear on specific locations in the body: the virus is most likely to originate where there are ganglions, globules of concentrated nerve cells in the body.

As the immunity drops, the virus replicates its DNA and increases the number of microorganisms around the nerve cells. The nerve cells are destroyed as the virus multiplies. The tiny nerves that are damaged are responsible for the function of the muscle fibers and skin sensation. The ganglions are located:

- in the head near the gland that requires autonomic nerve regulation, and
- along the spinal cord, on both sides, commanding the sensory bodies of the skin of torso.

The appearance of herpes zoster in the population of young people may indicate immunodeficiency, which leads doctors to perform various tests to exclude/prove the possibility of HIV, tumors, or other chronic conditions in younger people. If the HIV is a comorbid infection, the treatment will become more complex because a better outcome is expected if both are treated. HIV infection requires treatment with antiretroviral therapy and improving the immunological status, along with antiherpetic treatment.

Other medical problems, such as diabetes mellitus, tumors, and treatment with chemotherapy and radiation, also compromise the immune system. The task of medical doctors and the family, but especially of the patient himself, is to avoid any contact with other persons who have herpes zoster or varicella to prevent possible infection. Since diabetics have an increased risk of developing cardiovascular complications, such as stroke or a heart attack, there is an even higher risk for developing shingles infection if there are any of these occurrences in person's history. This is why it is also important to watch for thrombotic complications and to prevent those events. (3)

It is not common, but herpes zoster may appear in those with stable immunity. Among those people, herpes zoster is an infection that doesn't induce any complications and is more easily treated, at least in most cases. There is a small chance of developing disseminated herpes zoster. Postherpetic neuralgia may also develop, but the response to treatment is better than with other populations. In conclusion, it is important to improve the immune system and to protect those who are more vulnerable to this infection and many others in similar ways. This may be done with vaccination, which empowers immunological response in people without any underlying disease, and it is important to work on public immunity to protect those who can't receive vaccines. (4)

Chapter 2. Symptoms of shingles

Herpes zoster may hide in ganglions and from there it induces illness in specific locations of the body on the skin and subcutaneous tissue. These areas are sensitively innervated by the nerves where the host ganglion is located.

The ganglions are bulges of nerve cells that are connected to the nerves that come from the centers in the brain and spine and with the nerves that start from the ganglion to transport the impulses to induce some action or sensation. The virus is comfortably seated in the ganglions for years until a sudden trigger wakes it and induces its replication. There are several locations where the VZV may hide:

- Trigeminal ganglion at the base of the skull;
- Ganglions of other cranial nerves in the head and face, most commonly the facial ganglion; and
- Dorsal root ganglions of the spinal cord that lie on both sides of the spinal cord.

The VZV may spread through any of the nerves that start from the ganglions and end at the specific area of skin, inducing symptoms. Nerves arise from the ganglions to innervate specific regions, and bring specific sensory adaptations, depending on the location.

A person may at first complain about some unexplained sensations, numbness, tingling, burning, or pain on site until the skin lesions appear. These symptoms come from neurological damage. False nerve impulses for sensitivity are perceived by the brain. Other symptoms are generalized and include malaise, headaches, and flu-like symptoms. They might be falsely attributed to flu or another respiratory illness.

Skin changes are similar to those in chickenpox: there are red spots and blisters filled with clear fluid, which then becomes dense and filled with pus, only to turn into crust after a couple of days. The blisters may also fill with blood, and become red or brownish. The skin rash is limited to the specific area of the skin for which the affected nerve is responsible and it doesn't spread anywhere else. The skin rash is itchy, which is the usual reason for people to seek medical help. The itching may be very uncomfortable and persistent. The same clinical image is present in the varicella infection. These itchy blisters are characteristic of shingles and can't be easily misinterpreted as something else, especially when combined with other symptoms.

The sensations that appear are caused by the inflammation of the nerve layers after nerve damage caused when the virus began to multiply. The myelin, the outer nerve layer, is affected. It is normally responsible for spreading the action potential, a signal that is transmitted between nerve cells to inform the brain if there is damage to any part of the body. If it is damaged, there are some changes in the function of sensation. If the nerve becomes inflamed, the brain receives false sensations that there is some damage to the skin or a change of some kind that is perceived as itching, numbness, or tingling. The most uncomfortable symptom is, of course, the pain, which is neuropathic, meaning that it comes from the change in nerve function.

Types and localization of the herpes zoster

Trigeminal shingles (herpes zoster)

The trigeminal ganglion is located at the base of the skull, right in the center of the head, all the way inside and behind the ear canal and tympanic cavity. The trigeminal ganglion is a part of the 5th cranial nerve, from which begin the three branches: ophthalmic, maxillar and mandibular. The ganglion brings nerve fibers for each of these branches.

V1—ophthalmic branch

V2—maxillary branch

V3—mandibular branch

The ***ophthalmic region*** is the area of the face from the line of the hair to the root of the nose and laterally to the outer part of the eyes. The area of the whole forehead and frontal sinus is provided with sensitive branches from the ophthalmicus. ***Maxillary branch*** goes from the ganglion through the upper jaw and gives sensation to the middle part of the face, including the nose, cheeks, gums, and teeth. ***Mandibular branch*** brings muscle fibers and sensory fibers. The area it covers is the lower jaw, gums, and teeth, but also the part of the face in front and above the earlobe and the ear canal. The nerve that is responsible for the ear sensation receives the fibers from the otic ganglion, which is another place where the virus may be hidden. This ganglion provides fibers for the large salivatory parotid gland. The innervation of the nose, for example, is complex, which means that, if the nose is afflicted with a rash, it could mean that the affected branch is either ophthalmic or maxillar. The innervation of the ear, as previously mentioned, is also complex, with most of the innervation coming from the auriculotemporal nerve. Also, the facial nerve passes very closely near the outer ear canal, which may be how the rash and paralysis of facial muscles are connected.

Herpes zoster will always affect one side, which is typical, and easy to notice. Facial herpes zoster is an especially common location, affecting the trigeminal nerve and can sometimes be difficult to treat, since it may include the eye or ear or mouth, and is easily complicated by bacterial infection.

The Trigeminal Nerve

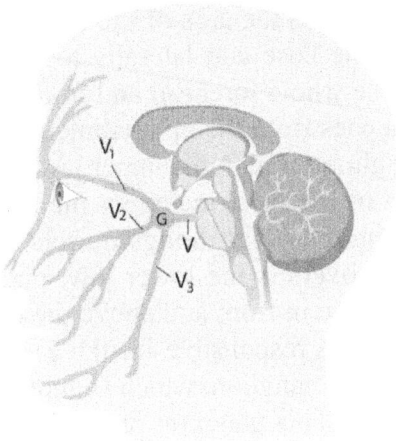

© Alila Medical Media - www.AlilaMedicalMedia.com

Figure 1. Trigeminal nerve and its branches and areas which the nerves cover

Any of these three branches or their sub-branches may be a pathway of the varicella zoster (VZ) virus.

Ophthalmic region

Ophthalmic shingles or herpes zoster appears when the ophthalmic branch of the trigeminal nerve is affected with the VZ virus. This type of shingles affects 10-20% of all people who have shingles. (5) When the virus affects this region, people usually have alarming and disturbing symptoms and are very worried, which is a natural response, because the virus affects the eye as well.

The symptoms include skin rash on one side of the forehead and pain in the structures of the eye and the skin around the eye. Depending on which sub-branch is affected, the symptoms can be more or less severe and differently located. The symptoms are:

- Severe pain on one side of the forehead, which may appear 1-2 days before the rash, and it may sometimes be falsely diagnosed as a migraine, a tension headache or sinusitis;
- Rash with blisters and crusts limited to the region of innervation of the certain nerve and that may or may not include the nasal area; and
- Eye symptoms such as red eye, pain in the eye, swelling of the eyelid, sensitivity to light, swelling of the cornea, blurry vision, or watery eyes.

The eye doesn't have to be included in the clinical picture, and the symptoms appear in about half of people with ophthalmic shingles. An indicator that inflammation is inside the eye is the appearance of a skin rash on the side of the nose, which is a warning and a sign that a person should definitely visit a doctor or even an ophthalmologist. Affected skin in the nose shows that there is nerve inflammation that spreads along the branches in the inner part of the nose and will eventually induce symptoms of an affected eye. There is a high risk for complications and the infection may spread inside the eye and cause vision damage and problems with eye pressure. The virus may affect the nerves of the cornea, causing it to become more sensitive to mechanical trauma and light, and forming small holes that damage the vision.

Therapy

Specific treatment of ophthalmic herpes zoster includes the use of the antiviral medication acyclovir and topical corticosteroids for the eye inflammation. They prevent further damage to the eye due to inflammatory processes. Corticosteroids are also used in some other illnesses of the eye where there is a high chance for development of synechiae and adhesions, due to excessive inflammation. The eye structures are tiny and fine, and any structural change may cause severe damage to the function of the whole organ. These excessive inflammatory consequences are reduced and controlled with the local application of corticosteroid hormones, in form of drops, for a limited period of time, usually 5-7 days.

Other medications that are needed if the deep structures of the eye are affected are pupil dilatators, which keep the pupil enlarged. This problem is also linked to the level of inflammatory response. If the adhesions attach to the borders of the iris, the pupil may become permanently constricted. That could lead to vision problems, increased eye pressure, other functional anomalies, etc.

If the eye pressure is increased, drops are required to reduce the eye pressure to a normal level, as a facilitator medication along with antiviral therapy. It is also recommended that the person uses analgesics to relieve the pain. If the analgesics are used when the pain is mild to moderate, it may prevent the progression of pain to a severe level.

Pain in the ophthalmic region may be very severe. This specific region induces very intolerable headaches. The pain is specifically treated with strong medications and some patients require narcotic analgesics. With time, a person will develop neuropathic pain, which is treated with specific medication that will be discussed later.

Maxillary region

The maxillary branch is rarely affected by the VZ virus. It is usually affected along with some other branch of the trigeminal nerve, most commonly the mandibular branch. The maxillary branch innervates not only the skin of the middle part of the face but also the inside of the mouth. Sometimes the first symptoms and signs appear in the hard palate, uvula, and/or tonsils and then they spread out on the skin of the upper jaw, lips, and cheeks. Sometimes, the eye is affected as well. The first symptoms are blisters, characteristic of varicella, which spread on the inner side of the mouth cavity, only on one side.

This rash comes in the form of blisters that can be filled with blood or as erosions covered with pseudomembranes (on the lips), that are formed analogously to the way the crusts are formed on the skin.

A person will in the first phase experience generalized symptoms, and then the symptoms will become more localized and will involve different sensations because of the inflammation of the nerves (burning, tingling, and itching). A rash in the mouth involves forms of ulcers after the blisters rupture. There could be only a couple of these ulcers, but they are very painful. These ulcers may easily be infected with bacteria. The symptoms and signs are always one-sided.

Treatment

The treatment includes antiviral medications (acyclovir), antibiotics in the form of tablets (systemic treatment), if there are signs of bacterial infection on the blisters as a complication, local anesthetics for the painful erosions and ulcers, calamine lotion against itching and skin irritations, and analgesics.

This type of herpes zoster can easily be complicated with secondary bacterial infections and severe pain in the palate, rarely in the nose as well. Some people have difficulties and pain during swallowing. This happens due to specific innervation in the mouth and inter-connections between the nerves. The nerves of the throat communicate with the nerves of the mouth. That is how the pain may spread to the back or cause functional problems. Proper treatment with antivirals, prescribed to be taken as systemic treatment, will help in these occurrences. (6)

Mandibular region

As in other forms of herpes zoster, symptoms are at first mild and generalized and last 1-2 days before other symptoms appear. The rash is in form of blisters on one side of the face, affecting the cheeks, chin and lower jaw, along the mandibular nerve of the trigeminus. The auriculotemporal nerve is a branch that arises from the mandibular nerve and, if it is affected by the virus, there is a possibility of symptoms in the ear. The eye may also be affected, but this happens only if there is also an infection in the upper branches of trigeminus. As with the maxillary nerve, there are blisters in the oral cavity and they too rupture and form painful ulcers. These blisters are in the mucosa of the lower jaw, underneath the tongue, and on one side of the tongue. The blisters are similar to those in maxillary herpes zoster, and are easily ruptured and become covered with pseudomembranes. The infection affects teeth as well, and they may become devitalized, because of the compromised circulation inside them.

Complications of mandibular herpes zoster include bacterial superinfections on the ulcers, prolonged pain, osteomyelitis (infection spreading to the bone), devitalization of teeth, and changes in the layers of the teeth crown. A person may experience teeth falling out and the resorption of the jaw bone; the bone may even become necrotic in severe cases.

Treatment

Treatment is similar to other types and includes antiviral systemic therapy (acyclovir, valacyclovir, famciclovir), analgesics, antibiotics, and, in severe cases, surgical intervention in the affected teeth or jaw, isolation, and treatment of the local skin and mucosal lesions (lotions, gauzes soaked in cold water). Corticosteroids are not recommended. (7)

Auriculotemporal region

The auriculotemporal nerve is a branch that arises from the mandibular nerve and is sometimes affected along with other parts of the trigeminal nerve. It is responsible for the innervation of the earlobe, ear canal and the region around it on the surface of the head, a temporal region. It may also include the jaw joint, the parotid gland, and the area behind the eye.

The symptoms begin similarly to other types of shingles: They are generalized and localized. A person may experience very severe pain that leads him/her to the doctor's office. When the herpes zoster virus or any other cause affects the auriculotemporal nerve, that syndrome is called auriculotemporal or Frey's syndrome and is differently manifested in children and babies than in adults. Usually, there is some swelling and rash on the skin with problems with salivation and tearing. Adults more often than babies have the interesting symptom of sweating while having a meal, which is a result of the false regeneration of the nerve branches from salivatory glands. This syndrome is, as previously mentioned, caused by many factors, usually surgeries and traumas, but it can also well e caused by herpes zoster virus. Children and babies only experience redness of skin and some swelling in the area of the salivatory glands, on the cheeks. Treatment isn't usually necessary if the sweating isn't excessive. In that case, the adults will receive treatment with aluminum chloride 20% or botulinum toxin injections or may require surgical intervention. (8)

This presentation isn't typical, and that is why it is mentioned here. It is rare, but it should be considered, among babies mostly.

Facial herpes zoster and Ramsay Hunt syndrome

Another name for this syndrome is herpes zoster oticus, and the ganglion that is affected is called the oticus ganglion. It is located near the ganglion of the trigeminal nerve. In herpes zoster oticus, the affected nerves are the 7th, the facial nerve, and the 8th, the vestibulocochlear nerve. The facial nerve arises from the brain stem and goes outwards through the temporal bone, passing near the outer ear canal, which makes it vulnerable to infections when the ear is inflamed. Those people who have had many ear infections in the past are at risk of developing Bell's palsy due to facial nerve affection. The facial nerve is responsible for innervation of the muscles of the face and facial expressions. When this nerve is inflamed and its function is damaged, it manifests as palsy or as a weakness of muscles of the face. Bell's palsy presents with asymmetry of the face and problems with eye closure; namely, the eyelid can't be closed and the eyeball rolls upwards as the muscles that move the eyeball normally do when the eyelid drops. This may lead to dryness of the surface of the eye and damage and fine scratches to the eye surface. This requires specific treatment and protection.

The 8th nerve follows the 7th most of the way and is responsible for hearing and balance. They both go through the middle of the skull, on its base, and enter a canal from the inside. Here the vestibulocochlear nerve is divided into two vestibular and one hearing nerve fiber. They then travel to the specific organs in the inner ear, and their smallest branches are for hearing and balance maintenance.

Sometimes other cranial nerves (5th, 6th, 9th and 10th) are affected as well, which makes the diagnosis altogether difficult. This happens because the pathways of these nerves are very close to each other and the infection is easily spread.

Ramsay Hunt syndrome includes pain in the ear, problems with balance, dizziness, buzzing in the ears, nausea, vomiting, involuntary eye movements, along with blisters and rash on the surface of the tongue but also in the ear canal and on the outer parts of the ear. It could lead to further symptoms and disorders such as hearing loss, headache, confusion, paralysis or weakness of the half of the face, which is mostly noticed around the mouth and eyes, and sometimes problems with closing the eyes. Problems with hearing appear in 50% of people, and in most of those people is transient.

The blisters can be seen from the outside and look similar to any other location. They may be filled with blood and crusts may form. Sometimes the blisters may become ulcerated and they may also become infected because hygiene is difficult to be managed in this area. The pain that arises in this form of herpes zoster may be unbearable.

This syndrome affects many parts of the face and may make prognosis in general difficult. Sometimes the paralysis appears a week before the skin symptoms, which may bring some difficulties with diagnosis because there aren't any obvious skin rashes that could indicate a herpes zoster infection.

Treatment

The treatment usually includes corticosteroids that decrease the excessive inflammatory response, B vitamins for recovery of the nerve fibers, eye protection (sometimes there is a need for covering the eye), physical therapy for facial movements and muscle strengthening, acyclovir (or valacyclovir) as a systemic treatment against viruses, local anesthetics and pain medications. Medication to treat vertigo, dizziness, and instability are welcome as well. Sometimes there is a need for a specialist's advice when there is structural damage to the fine ear organ parts.

Ramsey Hunt syndrome appears more frequently in the elderly. (9) However, there could is a possibility of complications that affect the eye or the hearing, which is why in most cases the illness should be taken seriously. Some people are left with severe pain even after the skin rash is gone. This pain needs to be adequately treated with specific treatment for neuropathic pain.

Herpes zoster of the skin of torso (dorsal spinal ganglions)

Herpes zoster appears very often on the skin of torso, affecting one side of the body. In fact, this is the commonest type of herpes zoster. The symptoms are similar to other types of herpes zoster, including generalized fever-like symptoms and blisters on the place of the affected dermatome of the nerve infected by the varicella zoster virus. The *dermatome* is the area innervated by one specific nerve, which provides sensations of warmth, cold, burn, pain, and itching. These nerves arise from ganglia that are placed on both sides of the spine and are actually globules of nerve cells. The nerves are called the spinal nerves. They are arranged by the parts of the body in which they are located:

- Cervical (lower back part of the head, neck, and shoulders);
- Thoracic (chest and back);
- Lumbar (lower back and abdomen); and
- Sacral (pelvic area).

Each area is divided into several segments in the shape of half-belts. The terms *shingles* and *zoster* actually come from a Latin word which means belt. These segments are known as dermatomes and only one segment and one nerve are affected by the shingles disease.

The rash and blisters form half of the belt: they spread from the spine to the front only to the midline and only on one side. The rash is at first reddish, but it later forms small blisters, then itchy blisters filled with fluid, which then collide into patches and crusts. These skin lesions may become infected, especially if the persons' immunity is severely impaired or due to false hygiene or the lack of hygiene. If the rash forms on the buttocks, it may be difficult to spot it, for a person himself or the doctor. Before the rash, a person will often complain of malaise, fever, diarrhea, or nausea.

A person also experiences pain that comes from infected nerves, which may appear before the blisters. This pain may seem very similar to some other types of pain, depending on its location, so the person may visit a doctor's office in the hope of finding out which inner organ is causing this pain. But this pain is also associated with other symptoms, such as numbness, tingling, itching, or burning. This is a sign that the pain may be neurological. However, before the rash, the doctors aren't exactly sure of the etiology, so they may perform some additional analyses before they conclude that it is, in fact, the herpes zoster infection.

The location of the rash is most usually on the lower line beneath the ribs, which is, along with the trigeminal area, the most commonly affected area with varicella zoster virus. The area is strictly margined and one-sided. The rash is similar to other types, except the blisters may be smaller and there may be fewer blisters with bloody content. Before the rash actually appears, the person may experience sensitivity to touch in this area. The rash appears differently to different people, but approximately 3-5 days after the pain had appeared. The rash will be present for the next 2-3 weeks. After the rash is gone, the skin on the site becomes hypopigmented (lighter than surrounding skin) and the pain remains for various periods of time. This may bring huge discomfort when the area is in contact with clothes. Even the slightest touch on the skin may induce great pain. This pain is called postherpetic neuralgia, which will soon be discussed.

There has been speculation about whether muscles of the trunk lose their functionality during and after herpes zoster infection of the same area, in the same way as Bell's palsy develops, but the data are insufficient. A consequence of such an event would be the formation of a pseudohernia (a hernia that doesn't include the intestines but only the muscles of the abdominal wall) and weak muscle reflexes. To check for any functional abnormality of the muscles, the doctor will probably recommend electromyoneurography.

Treatment

The treatment of this type of herpes zoster requires wiping with calming agents and keeping the skin clean, for example, boric acid 3%, or 5% aluminum acetate or sterile saline (five times a day for 30 minutes); powder for chickenpox, for example, zinc oxide with iron oxide (calamine lotion) against itching; acyclovir (or valacyclovir) locally or in form of tablets for those with low immunity; local or systemic antibiotics, analgesics, and treatment of pain. A normal level of hygiene is required. If the symptoms are resistant to conventional treatment, a doctor will consider alternative measures. (10)

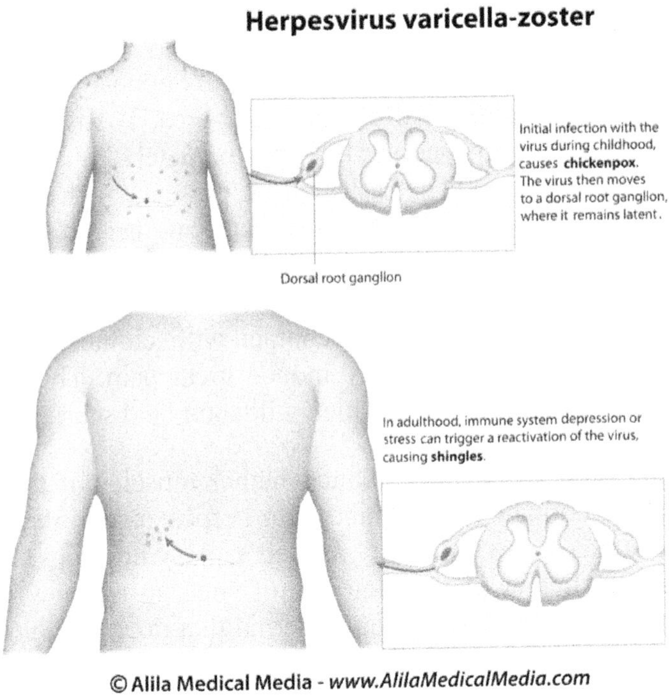

Herpesvirus varicella-zoster

Initial infection with the virus during childhood, causes **chickenpox**. The virus then moves to a dorsal root ganglion, where it remains latent.

Dorsal root ganglion

In adulthood, immune system depression or stress can trigger a reactivation of the virus, causing **shingles**.

© Alila Medical Media - www.AlilaMedicalMedia.com

Figure 2. The history and pathogenesis of chickenpox and shingles in the dorsal spinal ganglia

Other less common areas for shingles

Occipital shingles—upper neck (herpes occipito-collaris)

Herpes zoster may rarely appear in the area of the occipital nerves. The nerves that are affected in this type are the C2 spinal nerves from the cervical spinal dorsal ganglia. The rash appears on one side of the neck with typical nerve sensations before the rash appears. The pain is localized in the neck, with elements of a headache. The pain is one-sided and can involve the right ear and the left part of the throat. Sometimes this condition may look like an occipital neuralgia, a condition where occipital nerves are compressed by the muscles under tension, which induces numbness, pricking, tingling, and/or burning in the area of the back of the head and neck. When the rash appears, etiology of symptoms is clear. The treatment includes acyclovir or valacyclovir and corticosteroids. (11)

Glossopharyngeal and vagal herpes zoster

The glossopharyngeal nerve is the 9th cranial nerve and the vagus nerve is the 10th cranial nerve. They both arise from the lower parts of the brain stem, spread towards the throat to the front, and give branches for the soft palate, throat, tongue, and upper parts of the larynx. If these branches are affected, which usually happens when other cranial nerves are affected, there is pain and functional problems with swallowing and sensation of taste. The rash on the mucosa might not be as evident and usually appears on the upper parts of the larynx, which is only visible during indirect laryngoscopy. Treatment usually includes intravenous administration of antiviral medications. This is a complicated type of herpes zoster.

Unilateral herpes zoster on multiple dermatomes

As previously mentioned, zoster may appear on many locations at once. This may easily be missed at the time of diagnosis. There are examples in which a person has pain in the lower back and in the leg. Now, since there are many nerves in the lower back that exit the spinal cord to innervate the lower back, pelvis, and legs, the virus may affect the part that is responsible for more than one dermatome. If the skin isn't examined and checked, the diagnosis and treatment may be inadequate. This neuropathic pain responds better to anticonvulsives and antidepressives than to pain medications and corticosteroids.

Herpes zoster may spread to other dermatomes or it may appear affecting several dermatomes at the outset. This is an indication of severely impaired immunity.

Herpes zoster of the urinary bladder, bronchi, pleura or gastrointestinal system-herpes zoster of the inner organs

Bladder and bowel

Bladder symptoms are not rare in clinical praxis but are rarely thought about. Among people who have inner organ manifestations of herpes zoster, one-seventh have bladder problems in form of frequent urination, blood in the urine, and itching and pain during urination. Sometimes there can be some problems in the release of the urine and urinary retention. This type of herpes zoster is mostly present along with herpes zoster in the lower back. The nerves that control the bladder and also the functions of the ending part of the bowel are placed at the bottom of the spinal cord. If the sacral nerves are affected, there is a high chance that a person will experience some difficulties with the control over the bowel (constipation and bowel incontinence) and urine. In some cases, similarly to the rash that appears on the mucosa of the mouth, the blisters may form on the inner surface of the bladder, causing irritation of the bladder and frequent urination. Other forms of herpes zoster are neuritis and myelitis. In neuritis, there is a problem with urinary retention, and myelitis causes urinary incontinence and a rigid wall bladder. On the skin, the rash will usually appear on the buttock, in the same modality as herpes zoster of any location. The nerves that are affected are S2 to S4.

Treatment

If the diagnosis is set properly and in time, which actually happens rarely because of the unusual symptoms, prognosis and duration of the problems are shorter. The treatment consists of specific antiviral therapy. Sometimes there is a need for catheterization—placement of a temporary or permanent tube in the urinary system to facilitate urination. This type more often appears in the elderly, who have weaker immune system and may already have some other problems with urination and constipation. There is also the use of corticosteroids in order to decrease the inflammatory processes. When sudden urinary retention occurs, a doctor should always think first of the herpes zoster infection. He/she should also consider administering some medications that relax the urinary sphincter—alpha blockers, for example. (12)

Bronchi and pleura affected by herpes zoster

Herpes zoster bronchitis and pneumonia may develop in those who have severely damaged immunity systems. These are people who have been treated with chemotherapy and/or radiation or have some immunodeficiency, which allows the spreading of the virus to the pleura. Any unexplained pain during breathing with symptoms of respiratory infection, untreatable with conventional antibiotics and in an immunocompromised host, may be suspected of being caused by herpes zoster.

The treatment needs to be intensive and usually requires intravenous administration of antiviral therapy. (13)

Zoster sine herpete or shingles without rash

This type of shingles is very difficult to distinguish from all other illnesses because there is no characteristic sign of a rash. The illness begins with flu-like symptoms, followed by pain in the area of one dermatome of the affected nerve. Usually, the doctor will suspect that some nerve is being compressed, with some degenerative processes of the spine. If the nerve symptoms are caused by changes in the spinal joints and with muscles, the neurological symptoms usually appear on both sides, while herpes zoster only appears on one side. This allows us to easily distinguish these two.

Some people have problems with movement and experience some type of mild paralysis. Ramsey Hunt syndrome is often seen in these cases. This condition raises alarm and concern about some other illnesses, malignant and systemic. After many analyses that come back as negative, if the pain persists with all the characteristics of nerve inflammation, there is a suspicion of herpes zoster infection, which can be proven by the presence of antibodies in the blood tests. (14)

The suspicion is raised when there is some itching, tenderness, and pain on only one side of the body. This may look similar to other types of damage to the nerves, caused by local swelling and compression or injury, but none of them actually has the flu-like symptoms at the beginning of the illness. The accurate diagnosis is, however, only made with blood tests and immunological confirmation.

It is treated with intravenous systemic administration of acyclovir, but if the organism is severely immunocompromised, not even this type of treatment will help in recovery.

Complications of shingles and their treatment

Herpes zoster may progress into some other disorders that are more complicated to treat. This usually happens if the therapeutic methods haven't been performed or weren't sufficient, but sometimes it's because of the severely lowered immunity of people who suffer from illnesses such as carcinomas, leukemia, AIDS, or other immunocompromising illnesses. Each of the following complications requires its specific treatment once it appears. They can progress further into permanent damage to systems.

- Postherpetic neuralgia is a neurological disorder that persists even after the treatment and manifests with neuropathic pain, along with some other symptoms: itching, numbness, pricking, or burning. This is the most common complication that patients experience and the main reason why they seek doctor's advice. The pain may be transient or may be prolonged for as much as a year after the initial symptoms and rash. This complication requires specific types of medications, but it may be prevented with the treatment for neuropathic pain on time, in the acute phase.

- Ophthalmic herpes zoster and vision problems appear when the virus enters the inner organs of the eye and the inflammation damages the structures responsible for eye pressure regulation, vision, and clearance of the transparent structures (which then become denser with inflammatory substances that create collagenous fibers and disable transparency). This complication is treated with medications that decrease the immunological response. The immunological substances, the cytokines and chemokines, arrive at the site of inflammation and activate inflammatory cells in the surrounding area and induce swelling (accumulation of liquid with which the immunological cells arrive at the site of damage). The liquid component in the swollen tissue is at first clear, but with time becomes dense and filled with collagenous fibers. This is a complex way in which excessive response may be a problem in a normal body reaction to the herpes zoster (but also some other causes); that is why it is important to use immunosuppressants like corticosteroids. This treatment is applied locally due to many negative traits of its systemic administration. This complication is in many cases entrusted to an ophthalmologist, depending on the specific status of the eye. Another complication in the eyes is the appearance of blisters on the surface of the eye, which happens rarely, but requires attention.
- Deafness appears when the neurological structures of the 8th nerve are affected, damaging the transmission of signals into the brain-neurological deafness. It may be transient or, in some rare cases, permanent, which depends on the beginning of the proper treatment. It may appear along with facial palsy if the 7th nerve is affected. The structure that is damaged is the labyrinth. Deafness or problems with hearing develop when the blisters and crusts are present in the outer ear canal. These blisters may easily become infected because of the difficulty of cleaning and hampered hygiene.
- Bacterial infections appear because of poor hygiene of the skin blisters. Some people are falsely advised to not clean

the skin when having varicella or shingles, which then leads to the accumulation of bacteria on the skin whose integrity is lost. Another reason for secondary bacterial infection is inefficient treatment of herpes zoster, which further lowers the local immunity. Bacterial infections are recognized by redness around the blisters, increased pain, and pus in the blisters. The most dangerous bacterial infection is necrotizing fasciitis (the infection gets into the layers of subcutaneous tissue and spreads very fast, which occurs when immunity is weak, and the bacteria very virulent), and it may lead to toxic shock syndrome. Bacterial infections exacerbate the general state of the ill person.
- Encephalitis is an inflammation that spreads to the brain tissue and layers of the nerves inside the brain, which happens very rarely, as a complication of facial herpes zoster.
- Meningitis appears when the inflammation spreads on the brain's outer layers (meninges). Besides neurological symptoms, a person may experience vomiting. This too is a complication of exacerbated herpes zoster of the face.
- Pneumonia occurs if the inflammation spreads into the lungs, most likely in people who are immunocompromised, the elderly, and smokers. Pregnant women are also predisposed to develop lung complications.
- Hepatitis is an inflammation of the liver that appears mostly in immunocompromised people, but it is a rare complication. Symptoms include abdominal pain and fever. There have been some cases where the clinical symptoms weren't clear, and there is a high chance that the symptoms will be atypical until the liver goes into failure. This is linked to very immunocompromised conditions.
- Granulomatous angiitis is a zoster vasculopathy, an illness that includes blood vessels. This type of vasculopathy is predominant in the central nervous system. It usually

appears with hemiplegia and can be a very dangerous complication, because it can cause hemorrhage in the brain with symptoms of paralysis or, on the other hand, it can cause obstruction of small and large blood vessels, causing a lack of blood supply to the brain. This may lead to a stroke or the person may experience mild ischemic events the (brain is intermittently without supply with oxygen and nutrients), which are transitory and last for about 30-60 minutes. The range of symptoms that could develop may include problems with speech, vision, gait, memory, or concentration. Vasculopathy may also appear in any part of the body, including the spinal cord and extremities, which makes it difficult to diagnose herpes zoster on time. (15)

Neurological disorders of herpes zoster

Since varicella zoster is a neurotropic virus, it is expected that there would be many complications affecting the nervous system. They may be due to generalized immunological deficiency or nerve damage due to direct damage by the virus. With the replication of the virus in the nerve cells, those cells are damaged, tissue becomes microscopically necrotic, and the nerve layers are destroyed, all of which is followed by inflammation. Through the microscope, it is characteristic to see an accumulation of the immunological cells and glial cells, which are responsible for healing the nerves. A range of neurological conditions may appear atypically, i.e., without the characteristic rash. The diagnosis of such neurological disorders is then made after lumbar puncture and a presence of antibodies in the cerebral fluid.

The specific treatment for these neurological disorders is to administer antiviral medications through the vein, with supportive treatment to prevent the nerve and brain swelling.

- Zoster sine herpete is shingles with pain and mild or no signs on the skin that could indicate a herpes zoster

infection, but with neurological symptoms present on only one side of the body, as with all herpes zoster infections.
- Preherpetic neuralgia is pain that appears before the rash, and this condition usually indicates that there will be some other neurological complications, which is important if there is a chance to prevent them.
- Meningitis and meningoencephalitis are complications that develop when the inflammation spreads to the membranes of the brain. The symptoms are high fever, stiff neck, nausea, vomiting, sensitivity light, and a headache. If the condition progresses, a person may suffer seizures and loss of consciousness.
- Ramsay Hunt syndrome is a herpes zoster infection, previously mentioned, that affects the 7th and 8th cranial nerves and includes problems with hearing and balance, with possible muscle paralysis. The rash is present on the skin of the face, in the ear canal, and in the mouth. However, a small percentage of people have zoster without rash, which presents like Ramsey Hunt syndrome. In that case, the only way to prove the diagnosis is through blood test analyses.
- Polyneuritis cranialis following zoster is a condition in which there is inflammation of more than one nerve, which happens only occasionally, usually with the cranial nerves. In addition, shingles with rash may cross the boundaries of one dermatome, suggesting that there are two nerves affected. But shingles without rash may also present neurological symptoms in the areas of, for example, the 9th, 10th, or 11th nerve and cervical spinal dorsal roots.
- Cerebellitis sometimes appears as a complication of chickenpox in children. Cerebellitis is damage to the functioning of the cerebellum, the small brain. The children lose their sense of balance, they have tremor in the hands (this isn't necessary), and they develop a specific type of gait. It can appear with herpes zoster in the elderly, which isn't in any way linked to their

immunological status, but rather to the age when they first had chickenpox in childhood.
- Vasculopathy is a damage of the blood vessels, which is another condition that can appear as a reactivation of the virus without rash. The consequences of vasculopathy are reflected in the function of the central nervous system. The symptoms are weakness, drowsiness, headache, confusion, anorexia, damage to the eyes, and others.
- Myelopathy is a rare neurologic complication that can cause paralysis in the legs and possible problems with control over urination and stool. Myelopathy may occur with the acute herpes zoster or as a neurological condition caused by VZV, but without rash.
- Eye problems appear as a consequence of inflammation spreading to the structures inside the eye with damage to the eye pressure control and vision after the optical nerve and/or retina have been affected. There is also the possibility of paralysis of the nerves that allow the eyeball movements (3rd, 4th, and 6th nerves). Each of the nerves has a specific function, and inflammation of one of them leaves the eye in an unnatural position (looking outwards, downwards, with or without lowered eyelid, etc.). (14)
- Postherpetic neuralgia is the commonest neurologic disorder in people with shingles. Between 50% and 90% of the people who have shingles, according to some studies, will develop postherpetic neuralgia. The pain is neuropathic, meaning that it affects nerves, leading to changed function and pain without any reason and damage to the tissue.

Chapter 3. Neuralgia and postherpetic neuralgia

First, we need to consider what neuralgia is and how it develops. The function of nerves is to transmit signals from the periphery to the center, bringing the warning signs to trigger a reaction that will avoid further damage. Neuralgia is a term formed from two Greek words: *neuro*, meaning nerve, and *algos*, which means pain. There is another term, neuropathy, which is broader and includes, among others, neuralgia as a symptom (from *pathia*, meaning suffering or feeling).

Nerves may be damaged in several ways: through injury, inflammation, compression, or direct toxic effects. In this case, the nerves are injured with a viral infection that has a direct impact on the nerve function. The nerve fibers contain a nerve cell with branches that connect the nerve cells with each other. The branches are small except for one that is the longest; this is the one that carries out most of the neurotransmission. This branch is called the axon, and it has its layers, the myelin through which the electric signal passes from one cell to the other and to another by jumping from one section to the other. In infectious diseases like herpes zoster, these layers are infected and damaged and there is a direct effect on the nerve function: There is a change in the transmission of signals, which in the brain is perceived as the painful or itching or burning stimuli, all false sensations. There is no real damage to the tissue from which the nerves normally send signals to the brain, but rather it is that they themselves are injured and they do not function as they are supposed to. That is why a person has similar symptoms as if he/she has some type of injury to tissue. Neurons, or actually the layers, need a long time to fully heal, which is why the pain may persist up to a year after a herpes zoster infection. It is also a condition very difficult to treat since a doctor needs to find the correct medication that would provide effective results.

Postherpetic neuralgia

Postherpetic neuralgia is the most common complication of the herpes zoster infections, shingles, which appears because of the inflammation of the nerve fibers. If the neuropathic pain is present three months after the shingles, by definition, this is called postherpetic neuralgia.

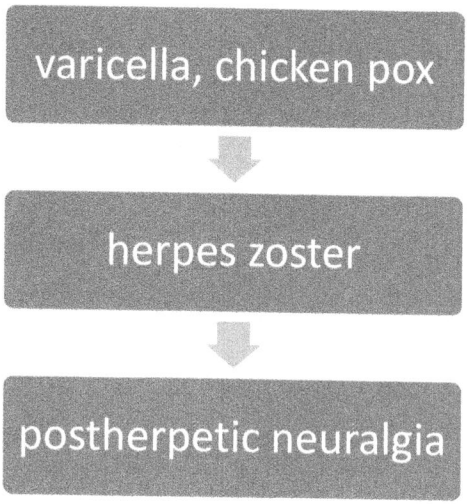

Figure 3. Order of the VZV viral infection and complications

Pathophysiology and theories of development

The herpes zoster virus is a neurotropic virus. This means that it has an affinity or a tendency to attack nerve cells. This may not be obvious when the chickenpox appears. However, after the chickenpox infection, the virus stays in the organism and hides in the nerves. Depending on which nerve is affected, we can have different regions with symptoms. Postherpetic neuralgia is considered not as a part of shingles infection, but rather a separate condition that requires specific attention and treatment. Still, the specific reasons why and how it appears remain unknown.

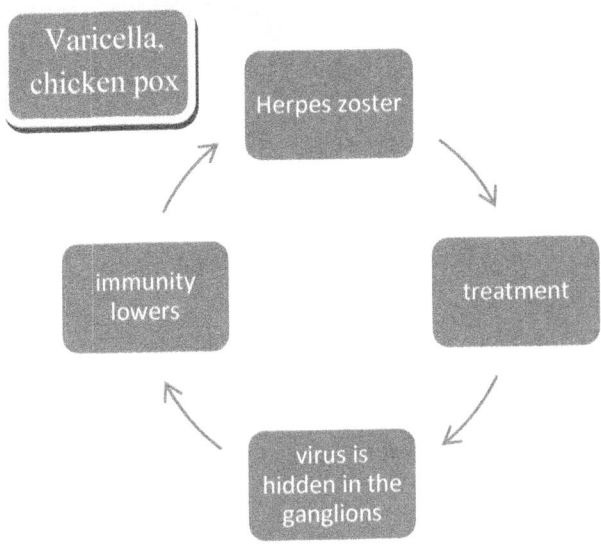

Figure 4. The cycle of the herpes zoster depending on the immunological state and treatment

Changes in the nerves develop because of the rapid spreading of the damage from the ganglia to the nerve cells proximally and distally towards the skin. If the changes become structural and not only functional, there will be some prolonged damage in the function as well, as long as the nerve doesn't get repaired. Sometimes when the changes are irreversible, postherpetic neuralgia occurs as a complication. (16) At least, according to one study, the changes are irreversible, but this should be taken with reserve. The effects of many medications with the action directed towards the transmission have shown great results and a complete resolution of symptoms, which may suggest that the nerve layers are highly regenerative tissue, and if the nerve cells themselves are damaged, some other nerve cells will re-form to replace their action.

There are some theories about how it develops. One theory is that, at the beginning of the shingles infection, there is so much damage to the nerve fibers that sensation is lost. There is structural damage to the spinal cord ganglions and neurons, which all spreads to the skin, which is affected by the loss of sensation and pain. Now, pain is a type of sensation, so how does it appear then? There are spontaneous amplified impulses that are transported to the brain from alternative pathways, when there is damage to the nerves that normally bring those impulses. These alternative pathway fibers are labeled Aß, and the damaged ones are C fibers. This is called *deafferentation*. This creates the continuous pain. Since Aß fibers normally transmit the signals for touch, and they have connected to the fibers for pain, now the touch will induce the sensation of pain. This is known as tactile allodynia. (17)

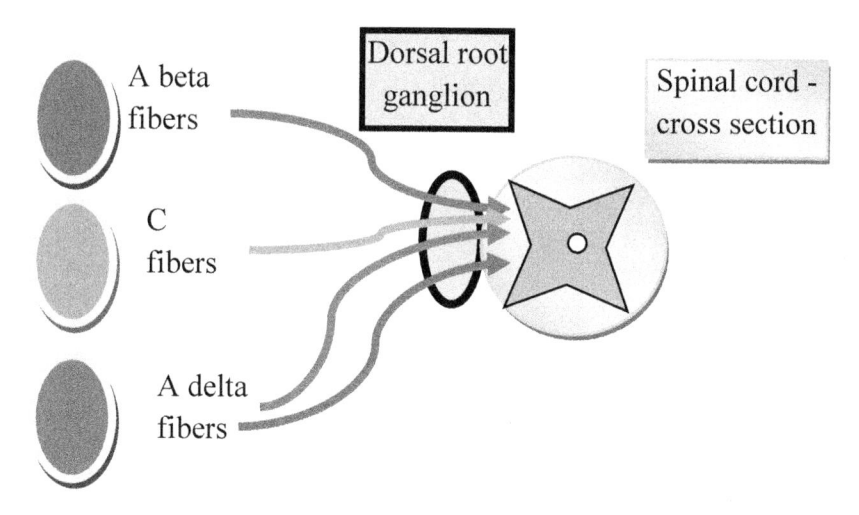

Figure 5. A beta, C and A delta fibers go through the dorsal root ganglion and then into the spinal cord.

Depending on the type of pain mechanism that dominates in pathophysiology, there can be three types of patients:

1. Abnormal functioning due to damage to the nerves that transmit pain stimuli, which presents with continuous pain;

2. Deafferentation with allodynia induces symptoms of sensory loss for hot and cold, but with pain on stimuli that aren't normally painful;
3. Deafferentation without allodynia appears because of the complete loss of sensation, so there is pain, activated by impulses from the brain, even though there is a complete loss of pain perception when pinpricking the area. (18)

Depending on the group, there are various therapeutic mechanisms that could help. According to this, the medications are programmed into specific schemes to have action on specific mechanisms to bring the most successful results.

Symptoms

In postherpetic neuralgia, there is some severe damage to pain perception and formation, and altogether there are several mechanisms from which the pain is generated. There may or may not be a lack of sensation to hot or cold or touch. However, pain may be divided into three categories, depending on the onset and characteristics:

Acute—pain present less than 30 days

Subacute—pain present between 30 and 120 days

Chronic—pain present more than 120 days (3 months).

Pain

Pain is either constant or it comes in the form of attacks, paroxysms. The pain in postherpetic neuralgia is described as burning, throbbing, cutting, stabbing, or electric shock-like. It may last for a couple of minutes and then diminish, only to reappear again, or it may be constant for several days.

It is usually worse during the night, which affects sleep. The pain may be perceived as superficial, as if coming from the skin and subcutis, or deep, as if coming from the inner organs, which may bring confusion to the diagnosis, especially if the rash isn't present. Pain reacts to the patient's psychological status, so it is worsened in situations of stress and anxiety, lack of sleep, or hunger. Pain may affect everyday life, including appetite and health in general. These patients often lose weight and feel tired and exhausted all the time.

Allodynia

Allodynia comes from *allo*, which means something foreign or other. Allodynia is a symptom in some neuralgias, for example, trigeminal neuralgia or occipital neuralgia. Allodynia is a phenomenon in which there is a sensation of pain when there shouldn't be.

The pain is triggered by otherwise painless activities, for example, dressing or touching the skin of the affected area. The fibers that are responsible are Aβ and C fibers. There is damage to the C fibers (and Aδ, as well, their function is similar to function and type of stimuli perceived by the C fibers). The Aβ fibers that transmit the impulses of pain become implicated in the perception of touch (tactile stimuli). This happens because there is a crossover of the impulses from the touch, perceived on the skin, that begin to travel through the pathways of pain to the brain centers for pain, and thus are perceived as pain. This is deafferentation. Nerve fibers lower their threshold as well, becoming more sensitive to stimuli, and they become spontaneously active. The area of skin is the starting point for neuralgia. Some studies showed that the amount of remaining nerve fiber endings in the skin may have something to do with the level of pain. Another factor is the warmth sensation perceived when another person touches the affected area.

There is also a theory of the protection of tissue. The role of pain perception is to send an alarm about the damage to the tissue. This pain is different, but still, the body protects itself from any outer stimuli, even the lightest ones, like a touch on the skin. This makes it nearly impossible to wear clothes on this part of the skin because it induces immediate pain.

Another theory suggests that there are no central inhibitory effects in neuropathy, which is why the stimuli reach the brain and the pain is created as an efferent response. (19)

There are three subcategories of allodynia in postherpetic neuralgia:

- Irritable nociceptor with allodynia, in which pain is severe and there is a problem with heat sensation with mechanical allodynia, which a pain that occurs in response to mechanical stimuli such as touch;
- Deafferentation with allodynia, which includes pain from normally painless activities; and
- Deafferentation without allodynia.

Allodynia is not present in all people with postherpetic neuralgia, but only in 50% of them. Allodynia is perceived differently in different neuralgias. The character of the pain and allodynia distinguishes them from each other. In trigeminal neuralgia, the pain that is provoked by otherwise painless activities is more shock-like and, in postherpetic neuralgia, the pain is perceived as burning-like. (20)

Unprovoked, constant pain

Pain may also be ***spontaneous and constant***, i.e., appearing without any factor that might induce it. The pain is burning, pricking, throbbing, and aching. It may appear intermittently with attacks of sharp pain. Even after the rash is gone, the pain in the area may persist with the same intensity. This type of pain can never be completely treated, but its intensity decreases until it is tolerable. This pain also affects the person's sleep and mood but reacts to anti-neuropathic medications.

Hyperalgesia and hypersensitivity

Pain and sensitivity appear because the nerves are meant to give an alarm if some destructive activity affects the tissue, when actually there is no damage to the tissue but rather to the nerve itself. There is a change in the nerve function. A person with this neuralgia also has a problem distinguishing hot from cold and experiences touch and a pinprick differently with changes of location of the stimuli.

The mechanism is a little different from allodynia: The threshold lowered in order to protect the tissue and because of the deafferentation of impulses. Increased perception of pain appears with painful activities, opposing to allodynia. There are:

-Primary hyperalgesia, which has a protective function and appears with damage of the tissue and the nerves' C fibers.

-Secondary hyperalgesia, which appears with the damage to the dorsal horn ganglions and is present without damage to the peripheral tissue. (21)

People with irritative nociceptors and deafferentation allodynia (the mechanism of allodynia previously described) experience allodynia along with constant unprovoked but amplified pain and pain from painless activities. The first group experiences heat allodynia along with mechanical allodynia, and the second group includes people with a loss of sensation in the area but the presence of allodynia and constant pain. Here, there is greater damage to the nerves. The third group doesn't include symptoms of allodynia but only complete sensory deficit.

Damage to the autonomic nervous system

The autonomic nervous system controls the function of glands and organs and has a role in other types of regulation that is out of our conscious and voluntary control. The nerves may control muscles, receive and transmit sensations, or, as in the autonomic nervous system, they may have different roles. If there is damage to the autonomic nervous system in herpes zoster, as an associated event, when the nerves and ganglions are damaged by the virus, it can manifest with sweating on an area of dermatome of the affected nerve or a change in the function of other glands. This is characteristic of the facial nerve herpes zoster. Some people experience abnormal skin temperature and color due to constriction or dilation of blood vessels on the region.

Some studies researched the effects of sympathetic nervous system stimulation in postherpetic neuralgia and acute herpes zoster. The sympathetic system is responsible for a "fight or flight" response and induces specific generalized involuntary actions like sweating, increased heart beat rate, constriction of blood vessels, and others. The studies researched retroactively with treatment that blocks the sympathetic system, and they demonstrated a temporary effect in pain relief, which is found to be insignificant in modern medicine. (21)

Zoster without rash

Pain may be reactivated in ***zoster sine herpete*** (previously described). This type of pain is explained as a neurological consequence of zoster infection. There is no evidence of the rash that might indicate a zoster infection, but there is pain that is persistent and restricted to one specific area on one side of the body only.

Musculoskeletal reaction

This appears as a protective mechanism and can be explained as an involuntary way of avoiding pain provocation. A person may put the arms in a specific position or make grimaces to avoid facial pain. There are signs of myofascial pain. This type of muscular pain is triggered by touch on close or distant points from the muscle. It is mediated by transmission of a stimulus through the membrane of the muscle. (22)

Another possible occurrence is mild paralysis of the facial muscles, known as Bell's palsy when the facial nerve is affected. There is a weakening of muscles on one side of the face with the inability to close one eye on that side, but with a lowered eyelid and erasure of the nasolabial groove. It can persist some time after the skin lesions vanish. This is why the treatment for nerve healing is important. The treatment includes vitamins and keeping the area protected from cold.

Psychological impact

Postherpetic neuralgia is followed by some complications that concern personal life and motivation. Some people whose skin lesions have vanished or are in convalescence don't quite understand the origin of pain or whether is it real. This may cause some problems with confidence or anxiety or some other psychosomatic symptoms.

Pain, no matter what the etiology, has a severe impact on our psyche. Pain may be acute and chronic. Chronic pain may induce problems in personal life and the quality of daily activities, especially if it is constantly present and doesn't diminish after the administration of analgesics. This pain is bothersome; it is always present and it appears with otherwise painless triggers, so people have to become more flexible with some activities so as not to provoke pain.

Pain disturbs daily activities and affects the mood, performance at work, patience in social interactions, motivation, and goals, induces emotional frustrations, and causes other problems, as well.

It can be the cause of mild to severe depression and anxiety disorders. Some people are already more vulnerable to depressive episodes, due to their family inheritance or personality or environmental factors. So, it isn't quite clear whether pain triggers depressive behavior in people who are susceptible, or the depression appears *de novo* because of the severity of pain. Depression itself may make the pain more severe. Depressive episodes may also be the reason why the shingles appeared in the first place. Depression is usually associated with some type of anxiety, nervousness, fear, and psychosomatic physical symptoms due to these. They may also increase the pain. This is why it is important to help these people, either with cognitive behavioral therapy and a similar approach individually or in groups or with the help of medications for depression and anxiety.

Pain that appears at night brings trouble with sleep, which may affect daily performance and concentration. Up to 82% of the people who suffer from any kind of pain have been diagnosed with insomnia. Also, sleep may influence the intensity of pain, with general fatigue, which also affects the psyche. Sleep deprivation may or may not be associated with depression and anxious thoughts. (23)

Chronic pain may bring general degradation of health, making an impact on physical abilities, social interactions, and psychological stability. Because of pain, a person may lose appetite and begin to lose weight and he/she may feel tired all the time and become less mobile. Some people may have so many difficulties that they require help in everyday functioning, which reduces their autonomy and increases their dependence on a close relative or a family member. This being said, the families may sometimes feel the struggles of a member who is in pain and has problems in functioning.

Epidemiology of postherpetic neuralgia. How many people with shingles will develop this type of pain and when?

Research shows that up to 1,000,000 people per year in the US have herpes zoster. The severity is different, depending on the immunological status of each individual. Only a part of this number will develop postherpetic neuralgia. (24)

Neuralgia may develop just before the rash along with other symptoms, but can also appear after the rash, which indicates that this occurrence is individual. Five weeks after the rash, nearly 30% of the victims complain about pain. Around 10% will develop neuropathic pain three months after shingles, and this percentage becomes lower as the time goes by. Pain is still present after one year in 3% of all people who had shingles.

There are still problems with zoster complications: The antiviral treatment needs to be begun in the first 72 hours after the rash appears but, in most cases, this doesn't happen. People don't notice the rash right away or they don't pay much attention and don't seek treatment. Many of them have said that they would surely act differently, and come to doctor's office sooner if they had known that proper treatment on time prevents complications. This counts especially for those who are immunocompromised. But sometimes the rash isn't one of the first symptoms. Instead, a person only experiences pain on one side. Many of the cases stay unnoticed by medical professionals and are treated at home. (25)

Risk factors

Some factors influence the condition: age of the person, gender, immunological status, some life habits, etc. Many of the factors have not been firmly connected with herpes zoster and postherpetic neuralgia. Some types of diseases are somehow connected with the chance that a person will develop neuralgia.

Age

The elderly have a higher chance of developing neuropathy, especially if they have a family history of the disorder. It is also understandable, from previous explanations, that people older than 65 have a progressive weakness of immunity and some researchers even believe that neuropathy is always present but with minimal manifestations in people older than 65. The dosage and virulence of the virus don't need to be high in order to induce nerve damage. With years, the myelin layer of the nerves is degrading and loses the ability to regenerate and reconstruct. As with other tissue, these layers degrade more or less progressively and become more vulnerable to a viral infection. This and the gradual decrease of the immunity are cofactors in the development of postherpetic neuralgia. Comorbidities increase the risk. Herpes zoster and postherpetic neuralgia appear very rarely in persons under the age of 40.

Gender

In some studies, women appeared to have a higher chance of having this complication, though many studies didn't confirm this. Two-thirds of all people with postherpetic neuralgia are female. The studies could be wrong, since among the elder population, there are more women than men (female expected lifespan is around 80 years, while in men, the lifespan is around 75 years), and there is another fact: women tend to seek medical help more often than men. However, women who go through the perimenopausal transition, are at higher risk for shingles and therefore also for postherpetic neuralgia. Hormonal alteration in that period of time and fluctuations of estrogen and progesterone affect cellular immunity. Hormones affect the whole body and their level decreases in the postmenopausal period, after the last menstrual bleeding. This also affects skin quality and density of bones, and may become a factor and a predisposition for many illnesses, not only herpes zoster and postherpetic neuralgia.

Immunological status and comorbidities

People who are immunocompromised generally have a higher likelihood of experiencing prolonged pain after shingles, especially those with diabetes (even though this illness is also followed by neuropathy caused by a high level of glucose in the blood) and illnesses that directly affect the immune system.

Other illnesses that might increase the chance for postherpetic neuralgia are kidney disease, rheumatoid arthritis, lupus, and inflammatory disease.

As previously explained, people with comorbidities, such as leukemia, cancer, or HIV/AIDS infections, have lower immunity, which is a direct factor in the development of herpes zoster and PHN. There is also a problem with the treatment of that illness that are associated with HZ and antivirals and other supportive treatment; for example, they might be interacting with each other, which can reduce the efficacy of treatment.

Psychological status as a comorbidity has shown significance in the risk of developing postherpetic neuralgia. Usually, people who have throughout life had problems with stress, somatoform disorders, anxious thoughts and behaviors will have a lower threshold for pain and show more worried behavior, which of course has to be respected by the medical professionals. They have to carefully approach the patient, convincing him/her about the pathophysiology of the neuro-psychological connection in neurological disorders, such as this neuralgia. Stress and anxiety could not be the cause of shingles, since the virus already lives in the body, hidden in the ganglions, but it may contribute to lowering the immunological status.

Severity of the shingles

If the shingles infection was severe and treatment wasn't efficient, there is a high chance that a person will also be confronted with neuropathic pain, which may be longer than in mild and moderate forms of shingles. If the pain appears early in the clinical picture, postherpetic neuralgia is a likely continuance of that pain.

Other factors

Smokers have a higher chance of developing postherpetic neuralgia, compared to non-smokers, according to some studies. This being mentioned, chronic bronchitis has also shown higher risk, without any evident connection. Having diabetes and being overweight or underweight were also included in the studies and have shown higher risk in people who were younger than 60. (26) (27) There is a need for further research, which will be important for prevention of the neuralgia.

Predilection places for postherpetic neuralgia

Some areas have a higher possibility of progressing into this complication. Two locations, the trigeminal nerve, especially the ophthalmic branch, and the chest region are the most susceptible for herpes zoster infection to be followed by postherpetic neuralgia. The pain is distributed as painful tics on one side of the face and, on the body, it presents as an amplified reaction to painful stimuli and pain triggered by otherwise painless activity. A person would often say that the clothes have suddenly become unbearable to wear and there is some itching and mild to moderate pain on one side.

Chapter 4. Diagnosis

Clinical exam

Taking a clinical exam and talking with a patient are starting points in your contact with your doctor. He/she will be interested to know when the pain and skin lesion first appeared. He/she may already have met with your condition. Postherpetic neuralgia is diagnosed when **the pain is still present after three months of the herpes zoster resolution**. You should also clarify which type of pain you have and how it has spread. The pain usually affects just one nerve in the same area where the rash was. If the nerve is one of the cranial nerves (in the head), there could be other symptoms or consequences to the herpes zoster, but if there was an appropriate treatment, these won't persist.

Symptoms and signs
- Severe burning pain
- Pain when touching, brushing on the skin, and wearing clothes
- Burning sensation on the skin with changes of temperature (hot or cold)
- Pain is overamplified with stimuli that wouldn't normally induce it with such intensity
- Itching
- Numbness or tingling
- Skin lesions hypopigmentation after herpes zoster
- Pain on restricted area of the body without rash
- Headaches if the shingles appeared on the face and head
- Sweating or abnormal reaction of blood vessels on site
- Bell's palsy
- Lack of sleep, insomnia, and fatigue
- Depression and anxiety.

He/she will be interested to know if you have any risk factors which would maybe worsen the prognosis of your neuralgia. These are conditions that lower your immunity, such as age and some other illnesses like diabetes, for example.

Neurological tests

Your doctor will probably check out the area where the pain is present. It is important to check for skin lesions, and to determine when they first appeared, if there were any flu-like symptoms, and if there was any pain during the prodromal period or when the rash appeared. He/she will touch the skin and ask you about what you feel and compare it to your sensations on the other side. He/she may perform a brushing test and you may or may not feel some burning sensations, which are unnatural for that type of stimulus. Sometimes, if the nerves are badly damaged, there will be no sensation. This is tested with pin pricking as a test for fine sensitivity.

He/she also has to check the muscle function and strength, because it is possible to develop a palsy and weakness during and after herpes zoster. This is specific for facial neuralgia. If the facial nerve is affected and Bell's palsy occurs, a person will have weakness in moving one side of the face, with possible salivation from the mouth, and problems with closing the eye on the same side. This may induce some damage to the eye surface.

Laboratory tests

Usually, the clinical appearance is sufficient for diagnosing postherpetic neuralgia. During chickenpox and herpes zoster, blood analyses can be used to prove that the virus causing the symptoms actually is varicella zoster virus. In acute infection, there are IgM antibodies in the blood and, if the infection happened more than four weeks before, your blood will show the presence of IgG antibodies for VZV. It is, however, difficult to accurately diagnose the onset of herpes zoster. High IgM usually indicates the reactivation of the virus, but only at the beginning of the infection. IgG rises for 10-14 days and, if the serology testing is performed in that moment, there would be no clear sign of reactivation, because IgG is also high before the infection, as a part of the immunological response from the first exposure to VZ virus.

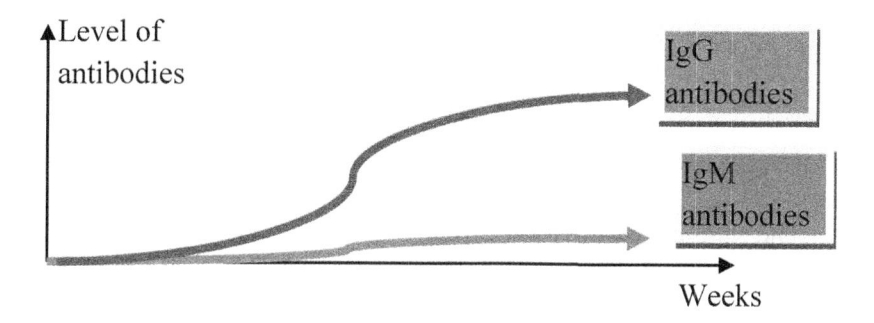

Figure 6. Level of antibodies during a VZV infection. If the IgM antibodies are increased, it means that there is an acute infection with VZV. IgG may be positive after vaccination and is not an accurate diagnostic marker if used alone.

When complications occur, especially in the brain, your doctor would have to order analyses of the brain fluid (cerebrospinal fluid, liquor) in search for different cell signs and viral DNA in it that indicate VZV infection.

Other diagnostic procedures for herpes zoster

Microscopic evaluation is not precise and may only indicate a herpes virus infection, without distinguishing between herpes simplex and varicella zoster virus. Tzanck smear is performed with a tool for scraping of the content from inside the blisters. This smear is observed under the microscope after it has been stained with Giemsa and, if characteristic multinucleated cells are found, it indicates a herpes infection.

DNA test, PCR (Polymerase chain reaction) is a more sensitive test for varicella zoster virus, but not available everywhere and very expensive. Another method that is very sensitive for VZV is *DFA (direct fluorescent antibody)* testing. (28)

Imaging studies

The use of MRI and CT scan is needed in neurological complications that may be present even during the neuralgia. (29)

Differential diagnosis

The diagnosis of postherpetic neuralgia is easy for a doctor. Usually, with information about previous skin rash on the site of the pain, the diagnosis is final. However, some conditions may look similar to it. They are:

- Trigeminal neuralgia,
- Cluster headache,
- Head injury or injury of the nerves,
- Hemifacial spasms,
- Persistent idiopathic facial pain,
- Migraine,
- Occipital neuralgia,
- Stroke and transitory ischemic event,
- Conjunctivitis,
- Glaucoma, increased pressure in the eye, higher than 21mmHg, which presents with severe pain in the eye,
- Trauma to the eye, foreign body in the eye, and damage to the eye, including keratitis and ulcers in the cornea,
- Vestibular neuronitis (inflammation of the sensory organ for balance),
- Sore throat due to infections of the respiratory tract (caused by Coxsackie virus, EBV, CMV, or adenovirus),
- Bell's palsy caused by other conditions,

- Heart diseases that present with pain (heart attack as the most severe one),
- Abdominal pain (gastric, pancreatic, gall bladder pain, appendicitis),
- Kidney stones and kidney pain,
- Infection of the urinary bladder (cystitis),
- Illness of the pleura, the membrane around the lungs,
- Back pain,
- Deformations of the vertebral column that compress nerves,
- Pain due to presence of tumors (mostly malignant),
- Psychosomatic pain.

Even the rash may look like something else:

- Atopic dermatitis with or without secondary bacterial infection because of itching and scratching, which damages the integrity of skin and allows the bacteria to enter and induce infection,
- Eczema or allergies,
- Contact dermatitis, after exposure to aggressive chemicals or plants with toxic effects; the clinical picture may range from redness to urticaria and blisters,
- Acne,
- Furuncles, which are infections of the skin that progressively affect the skin, hair follicles, and the surrounding subcutaneous soft tissue on the surface,
- Herpes simplex infection,
- Erysipelas, a Streptococcal infection of the skin with redness and swelling,
- Lichen planus, a condition that appears for unclear reasons, and manifests with itching, but the skin lesions appear on both sides of the body,
- Insect bites.

Chapter 5. Treatment

Through time, the therapeutic methods for pain have changed. With prolonged research, the aim of research changed as there were new theories about the pathophysiology of postherpetic pain.

First care for pain

At the very beginning of the shingles infection, there is a need to proceed with some therapeutic measures to assure that there will be a quick recovery and absence of complications, especially long-term neuropathic pain. Many people complain about irritability and pain when clothes rub on the skin. In this case, you should cover the skin with plastic wound dressing or a cling film and wear comfortable clothes that are made of natural materials. (30)

Cold compresses

Cold compresses are used to calm the itching and numb the nerves, which then decreases the pain. Aluminum acetate is sometimes applied to the skin lesions. In some cases, it could be uncomfortable to apply cold packs where the pain is and, in that case, you shouldn't use it.

Capsaicin creams and skin patch

Capsaicin is a substance that can be found in nature in peppers and is the reason why they are hot. Capsaicin has been used as a form of local treatment for neuralgia and some muscle injuries. Its main effects include dilatation of the blood vessels in the skin, providing more blood to the area and improving healing of the muscle fibers and nerves. In neuropathies, where nerves are damaged, there is a need for quick healing and blockage of pain.

Capsaicin has been used for a long time, at least 150 years, for treatment of various conditions that include persistent pain, itching, and burning sensations. It is produced as cream, patches, and lotions, diluted and sold as a 0.025–0.1% capsaicin product. It is applied 3-5 times a day for a period between two and six weeks. The effects will appear after continuous use of capsaicin for four weeks. The creams and lotions sometimes require gloves when applying or thorough hand washing after use. The creams induce burning sensations, which are very uncomfortable. Patches are made with 8-9% of capsaicin and applied directly to the area of aching skin. Capsaicin is, in all three types of application, minimally absorbed through the skin, and it works subcutaneously.

The mechanism of action of capsaicin products is on Substance P and calcitonin gene-related peptide. That has been the theory for a long time even though scientists don't think that it is the main mechanism. Namely, Substance P is known to be a mediator in the formation of pain sensation. This happens in inflammations, injuries, and other damage. Capsaicin has been proved to decrease the amount of Substance P at the site of the inflammation. Another mechanism that is possibly effective is the defunctionalization of the nerve fibers. What does this mean? It means that capsaicin blocks the sensation through the nerves on the periphery that are responsible for sensation. It also decreases skin hypersensitivity and hyperalgesia (lowered pain threshold). Capsaicin influences the way nerves communicate with each other, thereby lowering the transmission of the signals for pain, which is the desired effect in the treatment of pain.

Capsaicin in vegetables and other foods is used in order to improve flavor and it is not toxic in small dosages. Products containing capsaicin can be bought without a doctor's prescription. It is considered a safe medicament. However, there are some anticipated adverse effects. First of all, the hands should be thoroughly washed with water after application, because capsaicin induces intensive burning sensations, which limits its use. Sometimes the area of skin where the patch persisted becomes hyposensitive to damaging agents, which can lead to skin injury and inflammation. Some of the absorbed capsaicin may induce systemic effects, which happens rarely. (31)

Capsaicin shouldn't be used if there is a hypersensitivity or allergy to this medication. If you are pregnant or on any medication, you should ask your doctor about the use of capsaicin. It also shouldn't be used when the skin contains open wounds or is irritated or inflamed. Apply a small amount of cream or lotion and don't cover it. (32)

The effects of capsaicin are debatable. There are some studies that showed it had long-term effects, but new studies show that, after continuous use, there is only increased risk of adverse effects instead of effectiveness.

Lidocaine skin patch and lidocaine cream (Lidoderm)

Anesthetics have been known since the 19th century as agents that induce numbness and relieve pain. Anesthetics can be applied in the form of general, partial, spinal block, and local anesthesia. The term anesthesia comes from *an*, which means without or no and *esthesia*, which means sensation.

Lidocaine is used in dentistry as a local anesthetic. It can also be used for the treatment of localized pain, especially neuralgia and neuropathic pain. It mostly helps with allodynia. Lidocaine is usually used in the form of patches or sometimes gels that are applied to the affected skin. Studies that measured the effectiveness of lidocaine in postherpetic neuralgia showed that most of the people felt complete pain relief and some of them had experienced lowered intensity of pain. This shows great effectiveness. The patches are applied every 4 to 12 hours, depending on the level of pain.

Lidocaine functions as a blocker of the neurotransmission of pain signals. It works only on the surface of the skin, so there is a small chance of systemic adverse effects.

Lidocaine allergy is common in the human population, so before you begin to use it, you should probably check if you are allergic to it. The patches are applied on a painful area of intact and not irritated or inflamed skin and worn for between 12 and 24 hours. If the area is covered, the effects are better, which doesn't apply to capsaicin. The patches and gels contain 5% of lidocaine. (33)

Possible side effects are redness, irritation, swelling of the tissue, numbness, allergic reaction (local or, more seriously, systemic, the severest being anaphylactic shock), change of mood, tremor, vision problems, increased heartbeat rate, seizures, etc. (34)

EMLA cream

EMLA cream consists from 2,5% lidocaine and 2,5% prilocaine, and it should be applied 2–4 times a day. Even six hours after application, the pain decreases significantly. The cream is absorbed in one or two hours.

The area of skin on which the cream will be applied should be thoroughly cleaned and dried. The cream is applied in thin layers. It is not supposed to enter the eyes, nose, or mouth, or be applied on injured skin because it can damage these sensitive structures. Also, the area of skin will become numb to any stimuli after 1-2 hours, which is why it is important to pay attention to outer factors, scratching or hitting the area of skin.

Side effects are similar to lidocaine patches: redness, swelling, and rash are the most common. (35)

Analgesics

Analgesics in the form of tablets are, in many cases, the first line of treatment. At least, the people who experience pain would probably try to deal with pain by using some of the pain medication that they have at home. They, however, have a mechanism of action that is not suitable for treatment of neuropathy: they influence prostaglandins, the substances present on site of inflammation. This is the case with NSAID analgesics.

Opioid analgesics are used for very severe pain, which can't be managed differently.

NSAID

NSAID is an abbreviation for "non-steroid anti-inflammatory drugs." This is a large group of medications that are the most commonly used for pain. They are used for headaches, menstrual pain, abdominal pain, pain after an injury or a fracture, etc. Their mechanism of action has been already described. They can be used also as therapy for high fever, increased risk for thrombosis and heart attacks, etc. So, there are many uses for these medications, but we are interested in their effect on pain, and specifically on neuropathic pain.

In neuropathy, there is no accumulation of prostaglandins and other inflammatory substances. There is an accumulation of Substance P, which may be reduced with the use of a NSAID. However, the main problem in neuropathy is the altered function of nerves, meaning that they are triggering impulses about pain when there is no damage to the skin they are innervating.

The pathophysiology of herpes zoster or shingles is, however, complex, because there is damage to the skin and subcutaneous tissue, caused by VZ virus. If the pain persists after the lesions have healed, there is a problem with unstoppable triggering from the site of shingles to the brain. The true effects of NSAIDs are here limited.

Opioid analgesics

Opioid analgesics are powerful against severe to very severe pain. Their mechanism of action includes activation of opioid receptors in the brain, which are natural receptors for substances in the body that are responsible for elimination or deprivation of pain. There are three types of opioid receptors: μ, δ, and κ. The most important one is μ, and morphine, the powerful analgesic, has a major effect on this receptor. Activation of these receptors induces almost immediate pain relief by activating the receptors in the spine, dorsal horns. At the same time, opioids induce adverse effects, and some of them may be dangerous, which is why the use of these medications is strictly under control. Possible side effects are constricted pupil (miosis), vomiting, suppression of cough reflex, respiratory infections, respiratory distress, euphoria, sedation, constipation, constriction of the smooth muscles in the walls of gastrointestinal tract (which is why, if there is a bile stone in the gall bladder or bile ducts, there are absolute contraindications for use of opioids, since the stone can't pass further to the bowel).

Another characteristic of these medications is tolerance and addiction. With chronic use of these medications, receptors set the threshold higher and higher, which requires higher dosages and, with time, addiction also develops. Addiction means that if the treatment with opioids suddenly stops, a person will experience withdrawal syndrome ranging from severe to very severe, in the absence of the substance, which the body had got used to. Addiction is not only physical but psychological as well.

There are strong, moderate and weak opioids. Some of the opioids (narcotics) come from nature and some are synthetic.

Strong opioids:

- morphine
- methadone
- meperidine

Moderate opioids:

- codeine
- oxycodone

Weak opioids:

- propoxyphene, tramadol.

The opioids present many risks for any type of usage. However, some studies researched the effects of long-term treatment of postherpetic neuralgia with opioids, and discovered great efficacy, if the administration and dosages were adequately controlled. (36) When comparing antidepressants and opioids in the treatment of postherpetic neuralgia, the effects are nearly the same. Opioids proved to be effective in treating such intensive pain. Oxycodone, morphine, and methadone were used and compared to placebo, and showed great improvement and pain relief. However, the stronger the effect, the stronger are the adverse, unwanted effects. Sometimes opioids are combined with antidepressants in order to amplify the effects and to lower the dosages needed. (37)

Tramadol is a medication with strong opioid-like analgesia but it inhibits noradrenaline reuptake, which makes it similar to a combination of antidepressants and opioids. It is used for moderate to severe pain. Tramadol was used for six weeks in studies and brought great results to people with postherpetic neuralgia.

Opioids are not to be used with alcohol or sedatives (benzodiazepines), for they may induce respiratory depression. Persons with asthma or any other respiratory problem should avoid using opioids. This also goes for pregnant women and those are breastfeeding. People with kidney or liver disease should be careful when using opioids. Tramadol may induce serotonin syndrome, which appears with higher dosages or in combination with medications that increase serotonin level. The symptoms of increased serotonin in blood are restlessness, nervousness, redness of the face, diarrhea, dilated pupils, increased heartbeat rate, sweating, twitching of muscles, and confusion.

Ketamine and n-methyl-d-aspartate (NMDA) receptor antagonists

NMDA receptors are involved in the sensation of warmth and hypersensitivity, which may be important in warming pain in postherpetic neuralgia. Both of these medications have shown effectiveness against pain. Ketamine is known as an NMDA receptor antagonist. It may be administered as a continuous infusion for very severe pain, and it relieves the pain, as confirmed by many studies, but has significant side effects (problems with maintaining consciousness, hallucinations, nausea, fatigue, and dizziness). Its effects are better than the effects of morphine, a strong opioid analgesic. However, its side effects are too severe for it to be the first line of treatment.

There is a product that may be applied directly on the skin. It consists of 4% amitriptyline (antidepressive that works by increasing serotonin and norepinephrine levels) and 2% ketamine (local anesthetic) (AmiKet), and is much safer. AmiKet shows better results than gabapentin. This product brings huge pain relief and is favored by patients. It has some mild side effects that stay local because the medication doesn't absorb through the skin. At the moment, this cream is being researched, for its effectiveness and side effects, as a cream of 1%. The cream should be applied 4mL, twice a day. (38) (39)

Antidepressants

In the treatment of postherpetic neuralgia, the first medications that were ever used were tricyclic antidepressants. Through time, their effects were slowly replaced with modern medications that have fewer side effects and that are more efficient.

There are several types of antidepressants that may be used in the treatment of chronic pain.

- Tricyclic antidepressants (TCAs),
- Selective serotonin reuptake inhibitors (SSRIs),
- Selective norepinephrine and serotonin inhibitors (SNRIs).

Tricyclic antidepressants (TCAs)

Tricyclic antidepressants were named for their chemical structure of three rings of atoms. These medications were the first medications that were found to have antidepressive effects. After a short period of use, scientists discovered their possible effects on neuropathic pain. They had mild effects on other types of pain, which may have something to do with a psychological component. However, when it comes to neuropathic pain and its genesis, there are effects on more than the psyche. Namely, tricyclic antidepressants increase serotonin and norepinephrine levels and block acetylcholine, which is significant in the mechanism of blocking of the pain. TCAs are recommended as the first line of treatment for postherpetic neuralgia. They are also recommended for other types of neuropathy, for example, diabetic neuropathy. The dosages are lower than those needed for treatment of depression. The beginning dosages are between 10 and 25 mg before sleep. The dosages can be increased after approximately a week. The effects appear after a couple of weeks. Usually, there is a need for continuous use for 6-8 weeks before the effects of pain relief appear. They are effective, as previously mentioned, on combined problems. So if a person suffers from insomnia or depression due to pain, that will improve too.

Mostly used are amitriptyline (Elavil) and nortriptyline (Pamelor, Aventyl HCI).

Side effects appear due to anticholinergic effects:

- Dry mouth and eyes
- Blurry vision
- Retention of urine
- Constipation
- Sedation
- Hypotension and orthostatic hypotension (after changing the posture, i.e., when suddenly standing up from laying down)
- Toxicity on the heart
- Possibility of seizures
- Serotonin syndrome. (40)

Selective serotonin reuptake inhibitors (SSRI)

These medications are very effective in treatment of depression. However, some of them were found effective in the treatment of chronic pain, by maintaining the levels of serotonin, as a natural analgesic, in the body by blocking the reuptake and degradation of this chemical.

Medications such as paroxetine (Paxil) and fluoxetine (Sarafem, Prozac), are most commonly used in the treatment of neuropathic pain. They are modern in relation to tricyclic antidepressants and they have fewer side effects, which is why they are favored by patients. However, their effects are less than expected and lower than those in tricyclic antidepressant therapy.

Fluoxetine and paroxetine may induce some side effects:

- Confusion
- Difficulties with breathing
- Cold sweating
- Dizziness
- Chest pain
- Tachycardia (fast heart beat)
- Muscle pain. (41)

These medications are alternatives to other medications. The effects still need to be researched in order to find the right type and dosage of treatment of the neuropathic pain.

Selective norepinephrine and serotonin inhibitors

These medications have proven to be very efficient in the treatment of neuropathic pain. Their mechanism involves blocking the metabolism of norepinephrine and serotonin. However, the real reason that they help in neuropathic pain is not clear. It is true that people with chronic pain develop psychological depressive disorders, due to reduced quality of life, lack of motivation and willingness, and this may be a mechanism by which the symptoms are generally reduced after use of this medication.

These medications have already been proven in the therapy of diabetic neuropathy, where the damage is in the nerves caused by increased levels of blood sugar. By the same pathology, nerves are also damaged in herpes zoster, which could be a sign that the SSRI may work here as well.

The most commonly used medications in this group are duloxetine, venlafaxine, and milnacipran.

Duloxetine (Cymbalta) dosages are between 60mg and 120mg a day, usually divided into two doses. At the beginning, the dosages are usually lower; for example, the starting dose is 20-30mg a day, to be increased based on effects and adverse effects. Higher dosages are linked with worse adverse effects, especially nausea and vomiting. Duloxetine is indicated for diabetic neuropathy, but studies show positive results in other types of neuropathic treatment.

Similarly to SSRI, duloxetine has fewer side effects comparing to the TCAs, because it doesn't have a blocking effect on cholinergic receptors. Possible side effects are lesions to the liver (it is toxic to the liver), high blood pressure, and tachycardia. This is why it is important to measure blood pressure and once a month to do the laboratory tests for hepatogram (AST, ALT, GGT, and bilirubin).

Venlafaxine (Effexor XR) is an alternative to Duloxetine and is given if a person doesn't respond well to Duloxetine. At the beginning, the dosages are 37.5 to 75mg. Then, the dosages are increased up to 225mg a day.

Venlafaxine can also be responsible for higher blood pressure and faster heart beat, which are mild side effects. Most commonly, a person will experience nausea, constipation, dizziness, or a severe headache. (42)

Anticonvulsives

Anticonvulsives are today falsely named, as they are not used only for treating convulsions in epileptic seizures. They work by blocking the channels of calcium, which is necessary for the transmission of neurotransmitters and signals between nerves. Neurotransmitters travel from one neural cell to another via a sac, a vesicle, and as they enter the cell, the calcium mediates in the release of the content of the vesicle in the cytoplasm of the cell. The neurotransmitters can be exciting and activating or inhibitory, i.e. they lower the function of something. That being said, in epilepsy and in neuropathic pain, we need to inhibit this neurotransmission in order to block these impulses to the brain. In neuropathic pain, the impulses are unnecessarily sent to the brain to alarm the body about an injury to the tissue or nerves, when they actually signal pain on a site where the damage is not as large. That is precisely how we could stop the neuropathic pain.

These medications should instead be widely referred to as calcium channel alpha2 delta ligands. There are two main medications that can be used in postherpetic neuralgia, gabapentin and pregabalin.

Both of these medications contain the letters GABA, which stand for gamma amino butyric acid, which is a neurological inhibitory neurotransmitter. These medications work by lowering the excitatory neurotransmitters, glycine, glutamine, norepinephrine, and Substance P, and by promoting GABA, the neurotransmitter that lowers the level of excitation and impulse-sending into the brain. However, they do not act directly on GABA receptors.

The first line of treatment of neuropathic pain actually contains the anticonvulsives, pregabalin or gabapentin.

Gabapentin (Neurontin) is a medicine for neuropathic pain, first in the line of treatment and first to be prescribed of all anticonvulsives. Starting dosages may be around 200—300mg a day, but some studies evaluated the benefits and adverse effects in the dosages of 600mg, comparing it to those dosages, and concluded that the effects are similar and the adverse effects are the same. The dosages of 200-300mg would not reduce the unwanted effects, compared to 600mg, but the effect is greater with greater dosage. The dosage is gradually increased for 2-3 months until it reaches 3600mg per day. However, with an increase of the dosage, the metabolism and effectiveness change, because the bioavailability becomes lower with high dosages. That is why the dosage is only a half of that dose, which is 1800mg a day.

There are gabapentin products that slowly release this substance into the body, gradually increasing the dosage. This way the administration of medicine becomes easier. These medications are also useful when they are administered as soon as the antiviral treatment begins to prevent postherpetic neuralgia if it's possible. Studies showed that administering gabapentin with valacyclovir lowers the chance for the incidence of postherpetic neuralgia. After three months, the risk is 20%; after four and six months. the risk is lower. (43)

Most common side effects are mild and include dizziness, lightheadedness, sedation, anxiety, depression, weight gain, chest pain, cough, fever, shortness of breath, and restlessness.

Pregabalin (Lyrica) appeared some time after gabapentin entered neuropathic treatment. It is an S-enantiomer of 3-aminomethyl-5-methyl-hexanoic acid, which has pharmacological effects on the neurotransmission similar to gabapentin, where gabapentin is considered as its predecessor.

They have a similar mechanism of action. Both of them have shown good efficacy and fewer medication interactions than all the other medications, and are for that reasoned favored in treatment. Pregabalin also has to be adequately dosed. First dosages are between 50 and 75 mg and are gradually increased up to 300 to 600 mg a day. Compared to a placebo, pregabalin has shown significant improvements in pain relief.

Pregabalin has also some side effects, most commonly noted are dizziness, drowsiness, blurry vision, double vision, fatigue, weight gain, and dry mouth.

Both gabapentin and pregabalin are favored more than the tricyclic antidepressives for their benefits, and gabapentin has a lower cost. If the TCAs induce some adverse cardiovascular effects, especially coronary vascular diseases, where heart blood vessels may become compromised in bring blood supply to the heart muscle, it is indicated to enter gabapentin into the treatment. (44)

Pregabalin and gabapentin have some differences. Pregabalin has shown six times more effectiveness than gabapentin, according to some studies, but the side effects were more severe. The adverse effects of pregabalin, such as peripheral swelling, were raised as a factor for excluding pregabalin from treatment. Each of them has specific indications in which they bring more positive effects. For example, gabapentin has shown better results in the treatment of postherpetic neuralgia and some types of seizures. Opposed to that, pregabalin has been more useful in the treatment of diabetic neuropathy and fibromyalgia.

Sympathetic nerve blocks

The ways in which the sympathetic autonomic nervous system is responsible in the pathogenesis of pain is still unclear. There is a possibility that, when the nerve fibers are damaged somehow, the sympathetic nerve fibers that grow into and out of these damaged nerves produce mixed symptoms, with increased sweating and constriction of blood vessels on site. The sympathetic mediator is norepinephrine, and the tissue reacts to it, creating symptoms of allodynia and hyperalgesia. This was proven when in the same situation, sympathetic promotors were injected and more severe pain was induced. If the sympathetic nerves can be blocked, then it could relieve pain.

Nerve blocks are another way to relieve pain, with injections of local anesthetics directly into the nerve, which produces numbness and pain relief. Usually, the anesthetics that are used are bupivacaine 0.25% and lidocaine 1%. At the beginning, the injections are administered twice a week. In many cases, it is the praxis to combine local anesthetic injections with some oral prescribed medications, such as gabapentin or NSAID or opioid analgesics.

Most commonly these injections are performed when the pain and herpes zoster are in the chest. The nerves spread from the back to the front and are known as intercostal nerves. That is the site for the injections.

The procedure follows these steps:

- The site of injection depends on the location of pain; for postherpetic neuralgia of the dorsal spinal roots, the injection is made on the back;
- Relaxants and sedatives are given to decrease the hypersensitive reactions;
- The area that will be injected in needs preparation and cleaning, and after that a medical professional will inject the local anesthetic, superficially in the skin and subcutaneous tissue;
- To find the location of the ganglion, the professional will use fluoroscopy (live x-rays that are recorded) or x-rays; and inject a contrast that will show on x-rays where the ganglion is;
- The injection of anesthetics, slowly and carefully, while watching the vital signs;
- 20-30 minutes after the procedure, the patient may move the part of the body to check whether he/she feels the pain or not; the pain is supposed to be decreased, but significant effects would require repeated injections and time;
- After the procedure the patient may feel some warmth on site;

- Even though the patient needs observation and driving home, this is a safe procedure and a patient may go home afterward;
- The treatment is repeated, and effects last approximately three months.

In many studies, participants claimed moderate effectiveness after one month and after three months of follow-up, which means that pain wasn't completely reduced but it decreased significantly.

If the anesthetic is administered into the spinal layers, the effects are stronger, relieving the pain, but studies do not fully support the use of such treatment. The same is true of paravertebral injections (bupivacaine 0.5% 19ml and clonidine 150 µg ml^{-1}).

Side effects of sympathetic nerve blocks include rash, warm sensations, itching, soreness or pain on the site, bleeding, and also tachycardia, elevated blood sugar, and weight gain (in prolonged use). (45)

Injection of the local anesthetics

Similarly to the previously mentioned locally effective patches of anesthetics, the injections induce numbness and pain relief. Mostly, the practitioner will use bupivacaine or lidocaine in petrolatum/paraffinum ointment. These injections can't be performed continuously and have short-term effectiveness, which is why they are slowly being replaced by other procedures. Anesthetics may be injected along with corticosteroids to decrease the inflammation around the nerve. This way, the effects are slightly prolonged.

There aren't any side effects to this procedure, except allergies, pain, and tenderness on site. It is probably the most effective if the injections are given on time, or actually when a person has an acute episode of herpes zoster. Then postherpetic neuralgia may actually be prevented.

Radiofrequency ablation and pulsed radiofrequency lesioning

Radiofrequency procedures use radiofrequency waves to heat the tissue and destroy the nerves temporarily. This is a new method used in neuropathies and neuralgias to reduce pain. There is continuous and pulsed radiofrequency ablation. These methods are performed with the help of CT fluoroscopy to accurately locate the ganglion that is selected for treatment. Specific treatment for postherpetic neuralgia is required: in the thoracic region, for example, if the nerve affected by the virus is on level Th5, there is a need to also perform these procedures on levels above and beneath this region (so these regions are Th4 and Th6). The practitioner will know approximately where the nerve is. For the thoracic (chest) region, the nerve is placed between the ribs and is known as an intercostal nerve. Intercostal nerves, arteries, and veins always go on the lower margin of the rib. This is where the injection will take place, with care taken to avoid possible injury of an artery or vein. If the pain is in the lower back, and it is very resistant to any other possible treatment, the medical practitioner will sometimes decide to perform pulsed radiofrequency epidurally, i.e., in the spinal layer and not on the dorsal ganglion. These epidural procedures show effects of pain relief in many patients for up to a year. (46)

Continuous radiofrequency ablation

This procedure uses radiofrequency waves to induce destruction of the nerve with heat. The nerve is damaged and the signal can't be sent to the brain. The signals of pain and warmth, which are amplified in postherpetic neuralgia, are gone after the treatment.

Continuous radiofrequency treatment begins with positioning the patient and preparing him for the intervention. Usually, the person is set depending on the location of the pain, and the medical professional will most often set the patient to lie with back exposed. The site of the injection needs to be cleaned and the patient is relaxed with medical relaxants and sedatives. The procedure lasts 10 minutes with individual pulses that last 75 seconds each. On the area of skin where the needle will be inserted, there is a need for application of a local anesthetic, most commonly lidocaine. After a couple of minutes, the procedure may begin. Radiofrequency needles (actually tight tubes) are placed in specific places where the nerves are and through them a medical professional inserts electrodes a couple of millimeters into the tissue. The position of needles and electrodes is carefully monitored with fluoroscopy. Through the electrodes, the professional will enter an electrical current of small dosage. The current is administered with 5Hz frequency and with maximal temperature on the tissue of 42°C.

It is also recommended to apply a corticosteroid injection at the site to avoid an inflammatory response to electrical current. The procedure doesn't take long and doesn't change the day routine much, and the patient may return home but should avoid any physical strain and rest as much as possible. Some people complain about tenderness or mild pain on site after the procedure.

The procedure needs to be repeated and the effects usually appear after 2-3 weeks. These effects are temporary and, with time, the nerve will begin to regenerate, and if it "over-regenerates," it will grow a structure known as a neuroma, a mass over the nerve, made of glial cells, that compresses and alternates the function of the nerve.

Side effects include increased pain, numbness, redness, swelling, and allergic reactions.

Pulsed radiofrequency procedure in postherpetic neuralgia

Pulsed radiofrequency is also referred to as the cold procedure because it doesn't induce heat to induce pain relief but uses radiofrequency in another way instead. This procedure is modern, using continuous radiofrequency ablation and causing fewer side effects, and there is less chance for development of neuroma as a complication. The current is delivered in pulses that last 20 milliseconds with pauses of 480 milliseconds and the tissue is cooling down in that period, so it doesn't get damaged. Pulsed radiofrequency induces changes in the C fibers, previously mentioned, but these changes are subcellular and not structural, so the pain transmission is blocked.

Pulsed radiofrequency is not only used in the treatment of postherpetic neuralgia, but also in neck pain (cervicalgia), back pain (dorsalgia), and pain after major surgeries.

The procedure begins the same way. Here also the practitioner will clear the area of skin, apply the anesthetic, and, after a couple of minutes for the anesthetic to take effect, the cold radiofrequency procedure may begin. In many cases, herpes zoster affects the skin of the chest, so the targeted nerves are intercostal nerves, where the intervention is performed on the angle of the ribs and, in most cases, dorsal root ganglions, which proved to be more effective and which is performed on the patient's back. The needle enters a specific location, monitored with fluoroscopy, and then an electrical current is entered in pulses instead of continuously (two pulses are made per second). This prevents heating of the tissue. The goal is to alter the nerve's function and break the signals that travel to the brain and bring the sensation of pain. Some patients receive pain medications after the procedure to prevent post-intervention pain and to amplify the effectiveness of the treatment.

The effectiveness of pulsed radiofrequency is longer than in the continuous method (it ranges from 6 months till up to a year), which is comfortable for the patient. According to one detailed study, patients felt a lot better, they functioned better, improved their mental state and strength, and became more socially active. All of this is the evidence for the better quality of life after pulsed radiofrequency treatment. Its advantage is its safeness, particularly when performed on the chest since the needle goes through the angle of the ribs and avoids blood vessels that travel on the lower margin of each rib. This is important and prevents further complications if blood vessels get injured

This procedure may not be performed with high professional accuracy since the needle can't be held in a vertical position for as long as the procedure takes. Another risk is the possibility of puncturing the lung, which creates a pneumothorax, a condition in which air becomes trapped between the lungs and the ribcage.

When we compare these two procedures, each of them has its advantages and flaws. However, continuous radiofrequency procedure is used when the pain is in the face, and the illness affects facial nerves, mostly the trigeminal nerve. For chest pain, a medical professional would rather use the pulsed radiofrequency method. Both procedures are promising. They can also be used when all other methods have failed.

Surgical procedures:

Endoscopic (surgical) and chemical sympathectomy

It was already mentioned that, in postherpetic neuralgia and the damaged nerves that result, there are better chances for pain relief if the autonomic nervous system effects are reduced. These are sweating, dilation of blood vessels, and sensation of warmth. Some pains have this sympathetic component and are reactive to such treatments; this is known as sympathetically maintained pain. This means that the pain is constantly under the active control of adrenaline and the sympathetic nervous system. Your doctor will examine the area of skin and evaluate whether the sympathetic nervous system is affected, as well as the dorsal ganglion. In many cases, there is a lack of effect, but the initial procedures may be performed to assess the eventual effects.

Sympathectomy is much more radical procedure than sympathetic nerve block. In this procedure, a practitioner will use endoscopy, which is a procedure for diagnosis and treatment that works through the endoscope, a tube pushed through the cavities of the body and natural openings or openings artificially made by the surgeon. The tubes contain a light source and a camera that provides a better picture of the location where the procedure is being performed.

This procedure was particularly popular and innovative in the US in the 1990s. Through an endoscope, a surgeon could see the "unseen." There was the possibility of approaching structures deep in the body without damaging the body structures and without complications. Endoscopic sympathectomy was used to accurately find the sympathetic ganglions in the neck to reduce the sympathetic symptoms and pain. This procedure is performed today as well, in any case where the conventional treatment didn't bring good results.

Sympathetic blocks do not count as destructive measures and their effects last only for a short period of time. Another way of action on the sympathetic system is with chemical sympathectomy. In this procedure, the practitioner will use chemical substances that are known to decrease the activity of the sympathetic nervous system on a certain area of skin. These chemical substances are phenol and alcohol. These two substances are better researched in pain syndromes such as trigeminal neuralgia, where the cause of the pain is unclear, the pain is severe, and frequent injections are required to relieve the pain. In trigeminal neuralgia, the nerve sends impulses to the brain because of the imbalance of electrolytes or other non-specific reasons. When the trigeminal nerve is affected in postherpetic neuralgia and herpes zoster, there are benefits to chemical sympathectomy. Phenol and alcohol destroy the nerves and thus they block their function, which is the desired effect in postherpetic neuralgia. After a while, the nerve will heal and the pain will come back, usually after three to six months.

Endoscopic sympathectomy procedure is a newer method replacing the open surgery used years before, which contained a significant risk of complications and worse outcomes. Endoscopic procedures are minimally invasive, involving small openings which heal faster than the large ones, even up to 10-15 cm and using laser or stereotactic thermal interruptions to damage the sympathetic ganglia. Which of these procedures will be used is decided by the surgeon. Endoscopic sympathectomy usually requires two or even three tubes that are inserted in the body: one for the light and camera and one for the tools required for the procedure; the third is inserted for additional help when necessary. These tubes are placed to make the maximum visualization and accuracy in manipulating the instruments. They can be interchanged to allow the best position. The surgeon requires a specific position of patient, depending on the type and location of the pain. After anesthetizing the area he/she will cut incisions of 2cm for ports. Through these incisions, he/she will approach the chest cavity and search for the sympathetic trunks, without damaging the pleura (lung membrane) or any important blood vessel. The sympathetic nerves are then recognized and resected. This diminishes the function of the sympathetic nervous system in the pathophysiology of pain. To protect the lungs, the surgeon will deinflate one lung on the side. When the nerves are cut, the procedure may end. The lung must be reinflated. A surgeon will pull out the instruments and suture the incisions. The scars of the operation are small and will heal quickly, with less chance of complications than in open surgery. (47)

The effects of such treatment for pain are effective but temporary. Patients are usually relieved for six months, when the pain occurs again. These procedures are thus performed only in cases where other options are exhausted.

Side effects or possible risks of this procedure are:
- Damage to the lungs, causing problems with breathing, coughing, coughing blood (hemoptysis), accumulation of

air or blood in the chest cavity that could compress the lungs,
- Allergies to any of the material used in the procedure,
- Increased pain,
- Increased sweating,
- Horner syndrome, which appears when the intervention is performed in the upper part of the neck, which is rarely indicated. The syndrome includes constricted pupil, drooping eyelid and problems with sweating on the area around the eye,
- Influence on the heart beat.

Injections in the deep tissue

Injections to the spine-epidural injections

This method continues the subject of the nerve blocks. The injections are made around the spine, in the outer layer around the spine (the dura). The effectiveness of such a procedure has been confirmed by many studies. Some studies researched the possibility of preventing postherpetic neuralgia with a single injection in the dura in the acute phase of herpes zoster. The injection contained one ampule of corticosteroids, methylprednisolone (80mg), and one with local anesthetic, bupivacaine (20mg). A single shot, combined with proper treatment by antivirals and pain treatment, can decrease the chance of postherpetic neuralgia by 20 times. There are variations to this procedure, providing the best administration and distribution of the medical substances.

These injections need a guiding technique. It is usually performed with the help of x-rays to allow the surgeon to find the correct part of the epidural space. This may not be easy, and the procedure is not used on a wide area of the dura, because of the possible complications. Sometimes the results are felt one level higher or lower than where they were desired. This may be the weak spot of such a procedure.

Paravertebral injections

If the injections are administered alongside the vertebrae, the procedure is referred to as the paravertebral procedure (*para*, meaning beside, aside from). The studies proved that if the paravertebral injections of corticosteroids and local anesthetics are made in the acute phase of herpes zoster, the chance for development of postherpetic neuralgia is lowered by eight times. When the studies compared the effects of epidural and paravertebral injections, the conclusion was that the paravertebral injections given to a patient every 48 hours for weeks bring much better results than the epidural.

Paravertebral injections with a needle are procedures performed by a surgeon. First, the surgeon will have the patient assume a specific position for surgery, which is on the stomach, with the back exposed and area to be cleansed with disinfecting agent. Then, he/she will administer a local anesthetic under the skin to numb the area just beneath the skin and paravertebral muscles, where the needle will prick. Usually, he/she will use bupivacaine, whose effects will last for the next 12-18 hours. Sometimes, when the condition of the patient requires it, the surgery will be performed under general anesthesia. To follow the course of the needle, the surgeon will use ultrasound or fluoroscopy. He/she will insert the needle in the specific area between the ribs on the back. As the needle is inserted, he/she will inject the saline solution, which deflates the lung, and moves the pleura (lung membrane) away from the site of the procedure so that they won't be harmed. The needle is inserted 2.5-3cm away from the prominent parts of the spinal column, which avoids damage to these structures but also provides an adequate place where the nerves exit. The surgeon will carefully push the needle into the paravertebral space. He/she will know that the needle is in paravertebral space when a slight loss of resistance is felt. This is when the initial dosage of local anesthetics is going to be administered. The dosage is usually around 5ml of anesthetic. Bupivacaine has long-lasting effects, between 12 and 18 hours for the first injection. That is why the surgeon will most likely choose it.

There is a modality of injections in the paravertebral region using catheters. The procedure is performed similarly, the only difference being the catheter, which stays in position and allows daily administration of local anesthetics and continuous nerve block. Syringes are filled with 0,5% ropivacaine or bupivacaine. The catheter stays sealed with benzoin and taped with medical occlusive dressing. This continuous administration requires special conditions, and it is usually best for the patient to stay in the medical facility. There is an increased attention to hygiene, and the catheter shouldn't be moved. In severe pain, a surgeon may administer an infusion of anesthetic after proper evaluation of the general condition. The anesthetics he/she will then choose are ropivacaine 0.2% or bupivacaine 0.25%.

If there are no effects and pain relief after half an hour, that is an indication to remove the catheter. In this case, there is no use of such treatment. A patient may also experience lowering of blood pressure, which is also an indication for detaching the needle/catheter. (48) Other complications and risks include accumulation of air or blood in the space between the pleura and the chest wall, coughing, and pain. If a patient didn't know about allergy to the local anesthetic, there could be some allergic reactions that range from mild to severe.

However, if everything else is paid attention to and the insertion of the catheter goes well, the person will be pain-free for some period in the future, the period being individual and varying among people.

Intrathecal medication-direct effects on the brain surface

Intrathecal injections are applied in the liquor or cerebrospinal fluid. This liquid is present in the whole central nervous system: in the brain and in the spinal cord. Administration of any medicine intrathecally allows it to be better distributed into the brain when there is a need for immediate effect. This type of procedure was criticized for many years, and there are still doubts when it comes to this procedure. There were attempts to prove that the inflammation is in the dorsal root ganglions and that this could be treated with intrathecally administered methylprednisolone. This, however, brings a high risk of possible systemic reactions. Previously, in the treatment of postherpetic neuralgia, opioid analgesics were used for the treatment of pain. This may only be considered if the pain is unbearable. (49) But the dosages are actually smaller if the opioids are administered intrathecally. This means that there is a smaller chance for systemic adverse opioid effects, mainly sedation and drowsiness, and also difficulties with breathing. Sleepiness and sedation are the most common problems with opioid treatment, and most patients sleep for up to 18 hours a day during the period of taking opioid pills. Intrathecal treatment has proven to be more convenient.

Administration of methylprednisolone proved to be more harmful than beneficial. There is not only a large risk of systemic adverse corticosteroid effects (mentioned previously), but there is also a high chance that the covering layers of the brain might become infected, causing meningitis or arachnoiditis. If the site of injection is too low and damages the fine, hair-like endings of the spinal cord, called the cauda equina (*cauda equine,* horsetail in Latin), there is a chance that cauda equina syndrome will develop. Signs of cauda equina syndrome, which is an emergency condition, are:

- Difficulty with urination,
- Difficulty with stool discharge,
- Loss of sensation in the saddle area,
- Sexual dysfunction.

There is also a possibility of administering other pain medications such as baclofen, one of the drugs from the group of muscle relaxants. Baclofen is a GABA agonist, which means that it supports the blockage of impulses from the site of the neuralgia and thus may be helpful in its treatment. Baclofen may be injected in one act or continuously in an infusion. It is also chosen after other treatments have failed to improve pain. It is more efficient, according to some studies on patients, to inject baclofen in the form of individual injections, rather than in infusion, and the level of pain relief ranges up to 80%, which is an excellent result. (50)

The intrathecal approach may be more efficient than an epidural, according to studies. In this procedure, as well, there is a larger benefit if local anesthetics are given along with corticosteroids. The most commonly used anesthetic in this procedure is bupivacaine and the most commonly used corticosteroid hormone analog is methylprednisolone.

Risks and possible complications of this procedure include lowering of blood pressure, increased pain (which comes from irritation of the dorsal root ganglion), and allergic reactions. (51) The adverse effects may be due to the substance that was being administered intrathecally, or due to the intervention itself. After the procedure a person may develop:

- Headaches,
- Blood accumulation in the central canal of the spinal cord,
- Infections,
- Granulomatous masses,
- Problems with breathing,
- Neurotoxic effects due to nature of the substance, etc.

Steroid injections

Corticosteroid therapy was originally used for the treatment of inflammatory diseases with increased immunological reaction. Before that, scientists discovered its effects on natural immunological response. The corticosteroids lower the number of granulocytes and decrease inflammatory swelling. These effects were researched at the beginning of the 20th century. In the middle of the 20th century, corticosteroids were used in rheumatoid arthritis, and later injections of corticosteroid hormones were beginning to be used for pain in the joints in osteoarthritis (degenerative disease of the joints, which affects joints that were constantly pressured and overused during lifetime and with time the cartilage becomes dehydrated and prone to damage). (52)

The use of methylprednisolone, a medical formation of corticosteroid hormones for treatment of immunological diseases is the most popular among all corticosteroids. However, it raises the risk of potential systemic effects to the organism:

- High blood pressure,
- High blood sugar,
- Increased hair growth,
- Obesity,
- Bone loss,
- Stomach problems,
- Lowered immune system,
- Bleeding in the skin, etc.

Because of all this, many patients cannot be given corticosteroids: people with diabetes mellitus, hypertension, and kidney diseases.

Corticosteroids are used only as a preventive measure against postherpetic neuralgia. When they are administered with antivirals, they can prevent neuralgia for the next six months, because they reduce the area of inflamed tissue. Corticosteroids may be injected via epidural or paravertebral administration, while intrathecal administration is not recommended in many clinical praxes. It is only suggested if other ways of steroid administration didn't induce favorable effects. (53)

***

If we consider all three main types of injection: the injection of steroids, epidural injections, and paravertebral injections, we see that their effects are modest but useful in some patients. They are considered as an option where all others are exhausted. The way they are administered and the possible systemic negative effects are the main problems with these procedures and therefore they are not indicated everywhere.

Spinal cord stimulation (neurostimulation)

Spinal cord stimulation is done through a device implanted in the area of pain under the skin. This procedure has been constantly improving and developing since the 1960s, when it was first used.

The procedure begins when the surgeon/medical practitioner inserts a hollow needle into the area around the spine after a patient has been positioned and lies on his stomach, the area has been cleaned, and skin has been numbed with local anesthetics. Through this needle, a practitioner will insert leads. He may need to make small incisions so the leads will easily fit into the epidural space. To ensure that the needle is in the right place, he will use fluoroscopy (live image x-rays). These leads are actually wires through which a small intensity of electrical current will be administered. With these electrical impulses, we can control the neuro-electrical transmission, which is important for the management of pain and painful stimuli that are being sent to the brain. The leads are implanted in the area. They may be placed there temporarily or permanently. The practitioner will insert them and send the electrical current to check for the effects. If there is no favorable effect, the leads will be removed. To check if the electro stimulator relieves pain, he needs the patient to be awake. The leads will be placed on places that induce adequate pain relief. Then the leads and wires are fixed and a generator is implanted as well, usually in the buttocks, chest, or under the skin of the abdomen. The location of the generator is determined by agreement between the doctor and the patient. The implantation is performed under sedation. After this procedure, there are some postoperative symptoms that are expected, such as pain. Other risks and complications include bleeding, swelling, infections, and movement of the leads.

Some medications are not allowed to some patients, depending on how they metabolize in our bodies. They degrade and excrete through liver or kidneys. In people with liver or kidney disease, there are problems with adjusting dosages. When this is the case, it may be indicated to think of some alternative procedures like spinal cord stimulation. Other procedures that may be tried first are radiofrequency ablation and nerve blockages. This procedure may be tried for postherpetic neuralgia, but with limited expectations.

Physical treatment

Physical treatment includes passive and active exercises. Passive exercises are done with help of physical therapist. Active exercises are done by the patient himself. The benefits of such physical activities are in strengthening muscles and relieving stress.

Physical therapy with exercises (kinesitherapy) is especially beneficial in patients with postherpetic neuralgia, bringing them strength, motivation, and improved health in general. These exercises should be introduced to you by the physical therapist, who will know exactly what kind of exercises and how much effort you may give, without inducing counter-effects. Each patient is evaluated individually and, based on the patient's state of health and previous physical activity, he/she will be assigned types of exercises he/she can handle, and that will have the most positive effect.

There are three types of exercises for patients with postherpetic neuralgia:

- Aerobic exercises, which are land-based exercises, such as walking in place, running, and moving, with breathing exercises; of course, the effort is programmed according to the general condition and body physique; it is also

beneficial for the cardiovascular system, providing good circulation in the organs, and also in the peripheral muscle-skeletal system. Aerobic exercises may also be performed in the water, and these are called aquatic exercises. Exercising in water is a type of passive-active exercise because the effort is smaller than with active-active exercises but lower than when the physical therapist moves the parts of the body in passive exercises. This is why it is easier to do these exercises in the water.
- Strengthening is done through exercises for muscles programmed according to muscle mass; they include putting effort on muscles, which is higher than the muscle can normally handle. This effort is made through the lifting of weights or pushing through resistance, which induces destruction and regeneration, as well as enlargement of muscles; it helps in neuralgia by supporting the muscle-skeletal system. They may also be performed in the water. Aquatic exercises do not require as much effort and are much more acceptable to patients, especially if they are only beginning with physical therapy.
- Stretching is used for improving the mobility of joints and elasticity of the fibrous tissue fibers. If it is performed as a type of yoga, with breathing techniques and with an accent on relaxation, this type has an emotional effect on the patient, especially in those exhausted by the pain and sleeplessness.

Physical activity is altogether beneficial for patients with chronic pain and also with sleeping problems that accompany pain, and it may also help to prevent complications of other diseases. (54) When herpes zoster affects the facial nerve and paralysis occurs, there is also a need for specific treatment. Besides the treatment with vitamins and protection of the nerve, muscles need to be exercised to regain full power, as it was before the herpes zoster infection.

Percutaneous electrical nerve stimulation/transcutaneous electrical nerve stimulation

PENS/TENS are procedures that include stimulation of nerves, which is used in the treatment of pain, as a part of physical therapy. The mechanism by which this therapy works is to inhibit pain signals from the targeted nerves to the brain, block the signals that come to that nerve, and to promote body analgesics and increase their values. If a body's opioid analgesics are increased, the body is allowed to be healed, as are the nerves that were damaged by the virus. TENS and PENS work through the mechanism of gate control, which is a term for blockage of constant signals that come from C fibers, whose role is to transmit the signals for pain to the upper parts of the central nervous system. The impulses that come from the stimulator inhibit the signals and restart them, and thus a completely different signal arrives at the spinal cord, which removes the sensation of pain. This is all done with low voltage electrical current, passed through the electrodes through the skin.

Besides the analgesic effects, TENS and PENS also have effects on vomiting and nausea and on stimulation of blood flow through damaged areas with inflammation or those that need healing.

The procedure of implanting the PENS or TENS stimulator is not very complicated. Usually, the patient will receive a trial type of TENS, if he/she hasn't received that type of treatment before. This ensures that the effects will be carefully demonstrated and the treatment dismissed if there is no benefit or if there is an aggravation of symptoms. A percutaneous electrical nerve stimulator is placed through and under the skin, while a transcutaneous stimulator is placed on the skin surface. The electrodes, usually two of them, are placed on the area of the most intensive pain. The electrodes are connected to the machine, the generator. TENS procedure is performed at least five times a week (20-40Hz and 1-5 mA), depending on the severity of pain, and the treatment takes about 30 minutes. It is best to do these treatments for 3-4 weeks, to obtain the maximum effect. TENS uses new products, electrodes that stick to the skin and are disposable. If that is not an option, the electrodes are held to the skin with tape. A patient may place the electrodes on the skin once he/she has learned how to do it.

TENS has proven to be effective for people with postherpetic neuralgia. The complications are mild and the entire treatment is described as comfortable and tolerable. (55) The procedure is considered to be safe and is indicated in treatment of many conditions, such as chronic pain, neuropathies, low back pain, pain after surgery, and also when the problem lies in the inner organs: in the bladder (hyperactive bladder or incontinence), pain in the abdominal organs, such as the kidney, gall bladder pain due to the presence of stones, or nervous bowels. For neuralgia, it can also be used in combination with other therapeutic modalities, such as the medications pregabalin or gabapentin, in order to amplify the effects.

There are several ways of administering TENS, depending on the frequency, duration of impulses, and intensity of the electrical current:

1. Conventional TENS has a high frequency, between 40 and 150 Hz, short pulse duration, and low intensity. The effects usually are only short-term, as the current is being delivered, and then it substantially lowers. If the pain is mild, the patient will probably benefit from such a procedure. If the pain is moderate to severe, these low-intensity currents have to be administered every 30 minutes and the pads remain applied to the body. Conventional TENS aims at Aß fibers and not those fibers that transmit the pain signals. This way, altered ways of transmitting signals and avoiding stimulation of pain centers is crucial. Aß fibers are much thicker and they transmit high frequency impulses, which is why this current needs to have to have those characteristics. They

induce some muscle twitching as the electrical current is being delivered, which is a normal reaction.
2. Pulsed TENS has low intensity and high frequency and is released in short-period bursts. The effects are the same as in conventional TENS; it is actually considered as a type of conventional TENS.
3. Acupuncture-like TENS (AL TENS) has low frequency and high intensity and is held in reserve, in case a patient doesn't respond well to conventional TENS. This type of TENS stimulates Aδ fibers, which induces major muscle twitching, and which may be the reason that this procedure is uncomfortable.
4. Intense TENS, which uses high frequencies and high intensities, is administered for only short periods of time.

PENS is administered with a needle that is inserted into the subcutaneous tissue. The needle is placed near the nerve responsible for the pain, which is best evaluated by the health care provider. It will take a specific procedure that must be familiar to the physician who will perform it. The patient lies on the back or stomach, depending on where the pain is. The area needs to be numbed with a local anesthetic. After the skin has become insensitive to pain, the physician will insert the two needles that will be connected to the source of electrical current. Then a small dosage of electricity will be delivered through the needles over a period of 20-30 minutes, during which the patient lies still.

At first, PENS was a diagnostic tool for accurately locating nerves responsible for neuropathic pain. With time, both patients and physicians discovered that these stimulations can bring long-term pain relief, and that is when it began to be used for these purposes. TENS may be done at home after the patient has been instructed how to use and what not to do with the apparatus. (56)

Problems and risks with the use of PENS/TENS are rare. One of the most common adverse effects is irritated skin on site, especially with repeated interventions. It is present in nearly a third of all the patients. This usually happens when these procedures are done properly, and the skin becomes dry even though it has been covered in thin layer of special gel. The skin may also react to the tape that holds the electrodes on the skin. Other possible adverse effects are swelling, tenderness, sensitivity, and a small amount of bleeding on the site. (57)

TENS and PENS are not supposed to be used if the patient has a heart-implanted pacemaker, suffers from epilepsy, or is pregnant. The places where the electrodes are inserted should be ordered and advised by the health care provider and not the patient. There is a risk of possible complications if the electrodes are placed on the front part of the neck, in the mouth or another cavity, or on sensitive skin. Patients who have impaired sensation and cannot sense burning or damaging of skin, should not receive TENS because they won't be able to recognize the adverse effects of TENS on time before the skin becomes damaged.

Even though there are some precautions to be taken with this procedure it is considered as a mostly safe procedure that is minimally invasive and causes only mild discomfort to the patient. It is also advocated that it can be very useful in patients who are constantly in severe pain, instead of continuously administering tablets of analgesics that actually have many adverse effects, especially after long-term use.

Some people complain that the effects decline, which is not due to rising tolerance of the body to the TENS or PENS, but appears because the pain worsens or there are some technical problems with the apparatus.

**

The effectiveness of electrical nerve stimulation is excellent, even among patients with postherpetic neuralgia. The effectiveness is between 80% and 90%. By the way, these procedures are also used for muscle pain in the neck or back, pain in the inner organs, pain during menstrual bleeding, other types of neuropathy such as that caused by diabetes (nerves are damaged with increased blood sugar), and problems with the bladder due to nerve damage.

In many studies, the result was greater pain relief with PENS than with TENS, which can be explained by deeper involvement of the therapy than when placing on the skin. The skin has its integrity and resistance, which protect the whole body from many aggressive agents: viruses, bacteria, UV rays and sunlight, cold and warmth, electricity, etc. PENS is recommended to people with resistant and refractory pain. Both PENS and TENS reduce pain and lower the needs for analgesics, improve sleep, and feel much better overall.

Adjunctive treatment

Other approaches are yoga, tai chi chuan, biofeedback treatment, acupuncture, meditation, and breathing exercises.

- Yoga and yoga Nidra are relaxation methods known for many centuries and used in ancient times. Yoga Nidra is a type of yoga that provides a sleep-wake state, which provides maximum relaxation. It is performed when lying down on a special mattress with supports under the back. According to ancient belief, chi (body energy) flow is blocked in pain and that causes discomfort and frustrations. From a scientific point of view, any neurological disease is partially influenced by the psychological condition. The pain may be altered with depression and anxious thoughts. The fear of pain becoming unbearable and incurable will probably increase the pan. This may be individual, but it stands as a fact. Any method of relaxation that releases boundaries of anxious thoughts is welcome in the treatment of pain. So it is with yoga. Yoga exercises may be performed in any position, depending on what effect is expected and where the chi flow is blocked the most. It also includes some suggestive thoughts so, if you feel resistant to this, you should at least try and focus on what you want to accomplish. The integral part of yoga is the breathing exercises. Through breathing, the organism slows the heart rate and reduces the level of adrenaline that is circulating in the bloodstream. Slowly the predominance of the sympathetic over the parasympathetic system is lowered, which is the desired effect. With continuous stretching and breathing exercises recommended by the specialist, chronic pain may be improved at least slightly.

- Tai chi chuan is a form of ancient Chinese martial art that is nowadays used as a practice for relaxation. It comprises exercises with stretching and also pulling and pushing movements done in slow motion and with repetitive characteristics. This type of exercise is performed while standing up and moving the whole body. As with yoga, this technique suggests learning how to control the chi. Tai chi is best practiced outside, in fresh air, three times a week, for between 30 and 45 minutes, depending on schedule and physical possibilities.

- Biofeedback treatment requires coming to a health institution that is equipped with a biofeedback machine. The patient lies down and a specialist observes the results on the machine. The name of the technique describes the feedback it receives about internal events of the body: heart rate, blood pressure, breathing depth and frequency, and the state of blood vessels and muscles. The key of this technique is to learn to control inner organ events that can't be controlled voluntarily—at least not directly. With the guidance of the technician, who is educated about biofeedback, the patient can learn how to lower the threshold for pain and the reaction of the body to it—the sympathetic stimulation-fight or flight response in stress situations (from the autonomic nervous system, which was already discussed). The autonomic nervous system dominates the sympathetic system under stress and releases many substances that fight the new stressful situation, but also decrease healing and pain. Biofeedback

techniques work for unknown reasons and by an unknown mechanism. At least the precise mechanism is unknown. It, too, is a relaxation method, and it can be used as a facilitatory technique to learn how to do other relaxation methods that influence our breathing, heart rate, and blood pressure. If the electrodes that detect these parameters are mobile and if the patient has a biofeedback program installed on his/her computer, they may be performed at home, with consultations with a feedback expert from time to time. In the feedback therapy, there are:
- Proper breathing exercises,
- Muscle exercises with intermittent stretching and relaxing,
- Visualization and meditation.

Biofeedback may be used in some psychologic-neurologic diseases and also in anxiety, depression, chronic illnesses, and headaches.

- Meditation is a part of the Eastern tradition and way of living. It concentrates on gaining control over thoughts and remaining relaxed in difficult situations when practiced regularly. Meditation is practiced in a dark, calm environment, without disturbing sounds and lights, in a comfortable sitting or lying position, breathing naturally and through the nose with the use of abdominal muscles. Meditation is a crucial part of mindfulness techniques. The sessions of meditation last six weeks, with a gradual increase of length of the sessions, and need to be practiced at least once daily.

- Breathing exercises are beneficial in learning how to release negative energy and breathing naturally. The proper way of breathing is with the abdomen while sitting or standing straight. This breathing may be exercised on workdays, making a pause in a busy schedule: a two-time pause of 10 minutes for breathing exercise may improve functionality, concentration, and productivity. The best position is the vairochana posture (the position of the

Buddha figure). In this sitting position, the legs are crossed, the arms are relaxed and placed on the legs so that one palm is over the other; the head is held straight, slightly downwards, allowing the air to flow from the nose directly and straight to the lungs; the air is released through the mouth, after breathing with the abdomen. This way of breathing is the most functional, obtaining the optimal volume of air and oxygen that enters the lungs and contacts the small blood vessels. These breathing sessions reduce the level of stress and release from anxious thoughts and should be performed daily and regularly.

All of these are mindfulness techniques supported by medical science that improve chronic pain significantly but accompanied by other treatments with a specific mechanism of action (these all have a non-specific mechanism of action, but are more than welcome in medical science). Scientifically, these techniques detach a sensation of pain as a trouble that worsens the general condition, making a negative impact on the body, but rather percieving it as an alarming and useful sensation, with methods to increase the threshold for pain and to better cope with it. This is known as cognitive reappraisal. In studies, 65% of people with chronic pain demonstrated much a better condition and a decrease in pain. Their mood improved and there was a lower incidence of depressive thoughts, nervousness. and mood swings. Compared to the people who did not undergo such measures to reduce stress, those who did had better physical functioning after an eight-week protocol of meditation and other relaxation methods. (58) (59)

***

- Acupuncture/dry needling arises from ancient Chinese traditional medicine that originated over 2000 years ago. It is based on the position of acupoints or ashi points in our bodies where chi (body energy) is concentrated the most. These spots connect the most distant places in the body, which explains the effects if the acupuncture or acupressure are performed on one part of the body, but numb the pain in another part. Acupuncture is today performed in special centers by an acupuncturist. He inserts special, thin needles into the acupoints, depending on where the pain is and thus the nerves are stimulated. A Western method based on acupuncture and acupressure is dry needling, but they are not to be confused with one another. In dry needling, the spots where the needles are inserted are according to the anatomy and not the chi points of energy. With these needles, muscles are stimulated, predominantly the receptors of the fibers in the tendons of the muscles, thus inducing relaxation, which may help relieve problems associated with neuralgia. Dry needling includes only the use of needles and not local anesthetics or corticosteroids as a ''liquid'' component of the treatment, which is why it is referred to as ''dry'' procedure. A number of studies failed to confirm the positive effects of acupuncture in postherpetic neuralgia. There is a need for further research.

- Herbal treatment can be facilitatory if used along with other medications. Alone, it has limited effects. Herbs that have positive effects on the nervous system are: St John's wort (widely used in neuropsychological conditions because it calms the nerves), valerian (relaxation of the muscles, sedative, and analgesic), ginger (administered locally after proper preparation), capsaicin (in chili peppers, but only when prepared and then administered locally), passion flower (neuropsychological conditions like anxiety and pain), willow bark (works against pain, when it is present in the joints, lower back, works very similarly to NSAIDs), rosemary (prepared as oil, powerful analgesic), turmeric (prepared as tea decreases cholesterol, relieves pain and decreases the itching stimulus), German chamomile (for neuropsychological disorders, decreases stimulation of the nervous system, pain in the inner organs), lavender (prepared from the flower and oil, it is used for neuropsychological disorders, including neuralgia), eucalyptus (from leaves and oil, for herpetic lesions), toothache tree or Southern prickly ash (effective for pain), corydalis (used for treatment of nerve damage), Jamaican dogwood (there is insufficient evidence that it is effective for neuropathic pain and neuropsychological disorders), meadowsweet (effects are similar to aspirin, effective for pain)m and Kawa kawa (effective for neuropsychological disorders, sedative and relaxant). These herbs are prepared with the advice of experts in the form of teas or oils that are administered on the skin. It is best to consult with your doctor, and he/she will recommend the most effective remedies for you, individually. Oils are not to be applied on skin with lesions. (60)

- Massage treatment has been proven effective in treating neuropathic pain. Various types of massage can be used for neuralgia: massage with ice packs is especially welcomed in neuropathy since ice numbs the nerves and relieves pain. This type of massage may be performed three times a day. The person lies down and is surrounded with towels that will absorb water from the melting ice. Ice is applied on the painful area. The process lasts for 20 minutes, and pain relief lasts for another 3-4 hours. This may be performed at home, with ice made in the cup, and the cup is then used for massaging. The cup can be made from styrofoam, as a cone, with one part that goes on the cover of the cup to protect the hand from ice during the massage. The ice is applied to the skin and moved in circular motions. Direct contact between ice and skin is not recommended because it can damage the skin. Ice is better applied on a fabric, and the cold effect is then lowered. However, if the ice is moving on the skin, this isn't necessary, if the treatment lasts a short time, for about 10 minutes. Ice should also not be applied directly to the bony parts of the body. The area to which the ice is applied should as small as possible, to provide less adverse effects and stronger positive results. Ice should not be applied in illnesses that cause constriction of the blood vessels, such as scleroderma, Raynaud's phenomenon, acrocyanosis, paralysis, rheumatoid arthritis, allergic reactions to cold (cold agglutinins, allergies to cold). Conventional massage may be useful in providing relaxation, relief from anxiety, muscle tension, and sleep deprivation. If the whole body is under massage treatment, a person concentrates on the painless areas of the body. It is best for massage treatment to be received in a special massage center, with trained specialists. (61) (62)

Prognosis after treatment

Pain in postherpetic neuralgia may last as long as four to seven years, even with treatment. If the pain takes its natural course, it will undoubtedly last longer. With help of various treatments, and with prevention, quality of life and pain relief are possible resolutions. The perception of pain is individual, as is the length of convalescence. Pain may be described as none, mild, moderate, severe, or very severe. Some pains last a shorter time, some longer. Severe pains in people with decreased immunity will most likely be resistant to conventional treatment, and they require special treatment or some procedures that are somewhat risky and are not administered routinely in postherpetic neuralgia.

The key to treating pain is in the prevention of pain, which can be done successfully with proper in-time treatment of herpes lesions on the skin and the use of corticosteroids early in the disease. Prognosis is better in those with specific characteristics: being male, being younger, having stronger immunity, being given proper treatment, and showing a good reaction to treatment. The location of the dermatome affected by the herpes zoster is also important: sacral (lower back), chest and facial locations are more vulnerable to postherpetic neuralgia. Those with immunocompromising illnesses such as malignancy, HIV/AIDS, state after transplantation, diseases that require immunosuppressive, but also with increased blood pressure and diabetes mellitus have a higher chance of complications due to postherpetic neuralgia, and difficulty with treatment is expected. Depending on the severity of skin lesions, the pain will be more or less expressed. Some researchers tried to connect the number of vesicles and crusts on the skin with the likelihood of postherpetic pain but failed to do so, because the vesicles change their look after a short while.

In most cases, postherpetic neuralgia will last for about three months and then slowly diminish, never to appear again. These mild types of postherpetic neuralgia are responsive to antidepressives and anticonvulsives, which are in the first line of specific treatment.

Studies agree on the need for prevention and proper treatment within 72 hours, with cooperation from the patient. The best effects are achieved with pharmacological treatment along with another alternative treatment, and dietary and lifestyle changes.

Chapter 6. Prevention

Preventive measures

It is important to know whether shingles is contagious or not. For people who have already had chickenpox in childhood, being around people who have shingles is completely safe. The virus doesn't spread the same way as chickenpox does. However, people who have not received the vaccine and who have never had chickenpox should avoid contact with people with shingles, just in case. They are prone to developing varicella zoster infection, which could then be a mixture of clinical signs of both chickenpox and zoster with pain. Pregnant women, children, and immunocompromised people who have never had chickenpox are a susceptible group and should be protected from becoming infected.

The virus is isolated from skin lesions, blisters, and crusts, which contain the contagious material. The above-mentioned groups should avoid contact with people who are in the acute phase of herpes zoster.

Treatment of herpes zoster

Antiviral therapy

Treatment of herpes zoster includes these dosages:

- Acyclovir (Zovirax) in a dosage of 800mg tablets, five times a day over seven days, or
- Famciclovir (Famvir) in a dosage of 500mg tablets, three times a day over seven days, or
- Valacyclovir (Valtrex) in a dosage of 1000 mg tablets, three times a day during seven days or
- In severely immunocompromised patients, there is a need for more aggressive (meaning immediate) treatment with

antiviral treatment: Acyclovir can be administered into the vein, 10mg per 1kg of body weight, every 8 hours for seven days.

Corticosteroids

- Prednisone in form of tablets, 30mg, twice a day for the first seven days, then 15mg twice a day for the next seven days, and then 7.5mg twice a day for the last seven days.

Treatment of postherpetic neuralgia

- Capsaicin (Zostrix) 3-5 times a day,
- Lidocaine (Xylocaine) patches every 4 to 12 hours,
- Tricyclic antidepressants: Amitriptyline (Elavil) tablets, 10-25mg, dosages are gradually increased until reaching the dosage of optimal response; or nortriptyline (Pamelor) tablets, 10-25mg, dosages are gradually increased until the dosage of optimal response; or desipramine (Norpramin) tablets, 25mg and gradually increasing until the optimal dosage; or imipramine (Tofranil) tablets, 25mg and gradually increasing until the optimal dosage,
- Anticonvulsants phenytoin (Dilantin) tablets, 100-300mg a day, and increasing until the optimal dosage; or carbamazepine (Tegretol) tablets, 100g, and increasing until the optimal dosage; or gabapentin (Neurontin) tablets, 100-300mg, and gradually increasing until the optimal dosage. (63)

B12 vitamin and other vitamins

Supplementation with B12 vitamin is effective and obligatory in the successful treatment of herpes zoster. The B12 vitamin is necessary for regeneration of nerve fibers. B12 vitamin may be found in:

- Red meat, fish, seafood,
- Shellfish,

- Liver,
- Cheese (low-fat dairy),
- Eggs.

If the level of B12 in the body is sufficient, there is no need for injections of OHB, because all of the vitamin given would be excreted from the organism, and there won't be any use of it. If the level of B12 is low, there is a need for B12 injections every two days.

B complex vitamins may be useful since they are also necessary for nerve recovery. They may be given in the form of effervescent tablets.

Adenosine monophosphate (AMP) may be used as a preventive measure against postherpetic neuralgia. AMP is injected into the body, even though it is a substance naturally present in our body. Administering AMP in the form of tablets still requires some research. AMP is not recommended to people who already use carbamazepine.

Vitamin C is needed for regeneration of connective tissue and may be useful in faster healing, by promoting building up of the blood vessels around the nerves, which would provide more oxygen and supply of nutrients.

Vitamin E, an antioxidant, may be useful in altogether regenerative processes. It facilitates positive processes and decreases inflammation.

Local treatment of skin and lesions

Topical treatment with home remedies (at least) include application of ice packs, with or without a massage treatment, application of boric acid, baby powder against itching and neuropathic symptoms.

Vaccination

Vaccination provides good cellular or humoral (with antibodies) immunity and is an efficient way of immunization against many diseases. Vaccination and immunization are performed in state-controlled program and are given to a population of people who are most vulnerable to some illnesses. The same is true of children's diseases and the zoster vaccine. The first contact induces immunity of the organism. Another contact with a virus induces natural response of the host, which is amplified after immunization, so it is much stronger than before.

There is a vaccine against varicella zoster virus, Zostavex, which is built from a live virus but with modified and reduced virulence. Compared to chickenpox vaccine, this vaccine is more potent to induce a much stronger immunological response. The vaccination is performed with a short needle in the subcutaneous tissue of the upper arm.

When applied to the targeted population, it prevents herpes zoster in 50% of the cases and it also reduces the incidence of postherpetic neuralgia to 66% of cases.

The targeted population includes those older than 60 years. There is no need to ask and confirm that these people had smallpox in childhood or zoster infection. The vaccine is administered and usually protects for about four years. At 60 years, most people get the immunity against chickenpox, but the infection wasn't evident to everyone because of undetectable symptoms at the time.

Since people older than 60 have a high chance of becoming infected with influenza and pneumococcus, and they could develop serious complications due to their lower immunity, they should be vaccinated against these agents as well, and the vaccination and immunization can include all three of them, simultaneously. The effects of vaccine decline with the age of the population being vaccinated. The immunological status drops with years.

The only limitation is that this vaccine has not yet been funded for persons between the ages of 50 and 65, and all the costs need to be covered by a patient himself. (64) This has a practical meaning. Since the effects of immunization last four years, if given to patients in their 50s, immunity won't last when they are in the most vulnerable period of life for herpes zoster.

This vaccine has some adverse effects that are considered to be of low significance and appear rarely: redness, pain, or itching on site.

Vaccination isn't possible if the person is immunocompromised. Logically, the injection of the virus won't induce an immunological response and the infection will grow instead. However, some people, for example, those with HIV whose T cells are still at a high level, may receive this vaccine. Other illnesses that reduce immunity are some tumors, and the treatment against them, radiotherapy or chemotherapy; autoimmune illnesses that are being treated with corticosteroids, which lower the immunological response; and leukemia. Pregnancy is also a state that does not support vaccination, at least not in the first trimester.

If a person has had allergic reactions to any component of Zostavax, it is forbidden to administer such a product in their body. The substance that is often the reason for that prohibition is gelatin in the vaccine.

In the active phase of the zoster infection illness, immunization is also not indicated, and it is postponed. In fact, anyone in the acute onset stage of any disease should wait for recovery before receiving the zoster vaccine. Also, it should be noted that it isn't to be administered as a substitute for chickenpox vaccine for children.

Works Cited

1. **WHO.** *Weekly epidemiological record. Varicella and herpes zoster vaccines: WHO position paper.* Geneva : s.n., 2014.

2. **Albrecht MA, Hirsch MS, Mitty J,.** Epidemiology and pathogenesis of varicella-zoster virus infection: Herpes zoster. *Up to date.* [Online] 10 25, 2016. [Cited: 2 17, 2017.] http://www.uptodate.com/contents/epidemiology-and-pathogenesis-of-varicella-zoster-virus-infection-herpes-zoster.

3. *Chronic medical conditions as risk factors for herpes zoster.* **Joesoef RM, Harpaz R, Leung J, Bialek SR.** 2012, Mayo Clin Proc 87(10), pp. 961-7.

4. *Herpes zoster in the immunocompetent patient: management of post-herpetic neuralgia.* **RW, Johnson.** 2003, Herpes 10(2), pp. 38-45.

5. *Population-based study of herpes zoster and its sequelae.* **Ragozzino MW, Melton LJ 3rd, Kurland LT, Chu CP, Perry HO.** 1982, Medicine (Baltimore) 61(5), pp. 310-6.

6. **Maassen J, Oetting T.** Herpes Zoster Post-herpetic Neuralgia:68-year-old male with decreased vision. *WebEye.* [Online] 2005. [Cited: 2 18, 2017.] http://webeye.ophth.uiowa.edu/eyeforum/cases/41-Herpes-Zoster-Post-Herpetic-Neuralgia.htm.

7. *Herpes zoster of the trigeminal nerve third branch: a case report and review of the literature.* **Tidwell E, Hutson B, Burkhart N, Gutmann JL, Ellis CD.** 1999, International Endodontic Journal 32, pp. 61-6.

8. **Gomathy S.** Auriculotemporal nerve syndrome / Frey syndrome/Gustatory sweating. *Pediatric news.* [Online] [Cited: 2 24, 2017.] http://www.mdedge.com/pediatricnews/dsm/11162/dermatology/auriculotemporal-nerve-syndrome/frey-syndrome/gustatory-sweating.

9. Ramsay Hunt syndrome. *Mayo Clinic.* [Online] [Cited: 2 24, 2017.] http://www.mayoclinic.org/diseases-conditions/ramsay-hunt-syndrome/symptoms-causes/dxc-20257240.

10. **CK., Janniger.** Herpes Zoster Treatment & Management. *Medscape.* [Online] 6 16, 2016. [Cited: 2 25, 2017.] http://emedicine.medscape.com/article/1132465-treatment#d7.

11. *Unusual Manifestation of Herpes Zoster Infection Involving the Greater, Lesser Occipital and Transverse Cervical Nerve: A Case Report.* **al., Mevio E et.** 2015, J Otolaryngol Rhinol 1:1.

12. *Sacral Herpes Zoster Associated with Voiding Dysfunction in a Young Patient with Scrub Typhus.* **J., Hur.** 2015, Infection & Chemotherapy 47(2), pp. 133-6.

13. *Cytology of pleural effusion associated with disseminated infection caused by varicella-zoster virus in an immunocompromised patient. A case report.* **Mori M, Imamura Y, Maegawa H, Yoshida H, Naiki H, Fukuda M.** 2003, Acta Cytol 47(3), pp. 480-4.

14. *Neurological Disease Produced by Varicella Zoster Virus Reactivation Without Rash.* **Gilden D, Cohrs RJ, Mahalingam R, Nagel MA.** 2010, Curr Top Microbiol Immunol 342, pp. 243-53.

15. *Varicella zoster virus vasculopathies: diverse clinical manifestations, laboratory features, pathogenesis, and treatment.*

Gilden D, Cohrs RJ, Mahalingam R, Nagel MA. 2009, Lancet neurology 8(8), p. 731. .

16. *Pathophysiology of postherpetic neuralgia:towards a rational treatment.* **D., Bowaher.** 1995, Neurology 45 Suppl (8), pp. 56-7.

17. *Mechanisms of postherpetic neuralgia--we are hot on the scent.* **R., Baron.** 2008, Pain 140(3), pp. 395-6.

18. *Is post herpetic neuralgia more than one disorder?* **Rowbotham MC, Peterson KL, Fields HL.** 1998, Pain Forum vol. 7, pp. 231-7.

19. *The relationship of pain, allodynia and thermal sensation in post-herpetic neuralgia.* **Rowbotham MC, Fields HL.** 1996, Brain 119 , pp. 347-54.

20. *A Novel Case of Resolved Postherpetic Neuralgia with Subsequent Development of Trigeminal Neuralgia: A Case Report and Review of the Literature.* **Mason A, Ayres K, Burneikiene S, Villavicencio AT,Nelson EL, Rajpal S.** 2013, Case Reports in Medicine, Article ID 398513, 3 pages.

21. *The role of sympathetic nerve blocks in herpes zoster and post herpetic neuralgia.* **Christopher L.Wu, Ann Marsh, Robert H Dworkin.** 2000, Pain, 87, pp. 121-9.

22. **Thakur R, Kent JL, Divorkin BH.** *Herpes Zoster and Postherpetic Neuralgia.* s.l. : Lippincott,Williams & Wilkins, 2010. pp. 338-57.

23. *Self-reported sleep and mood disturbance in chronic pain patients.* **Morin CM, Gibson D, Wade J.** 1998, Clin J Pain. 14(4), pp. 311-4.

24. *A population-based study of the incidence and complication rates of herpes zoster before zoster vaccine introduction.* **Yawn BP, Saddier P, Wollan P, St. Sauver JL, Kurland MJ, Sy LS.** 2007, Mayo Clin Proc 82, pp. 1341-9.

25. *Consequences and Management of Pain in Herpes Zoster .* **RW., Johnson.** 2002, J Infect Dis 186(1), pp. 83-90 .

26. *Quantification of risk factors for postherpetic neuralgia in herpes zoster patients: A cohort study.* **Forbes HJ, Bhaskaran K, Thomas SL, et al.** 2016, Neurology 87(1), pp. 94-102.

27. *Post-herpetic neuralgia .* **Gupta R, Smith PF.** 2012, Contin Educ Anaesth Crit Care Pain 12(4) , pp. 181-5.

28. **CK., Janniger.** Herpes Zoster Workup. *Emedicine Medscape.* [Online] [Cited: 3 25, 2017.] http://emedicine.medscape.com/article/1132465-workup#c6.

29. *CSF and MRI findings in patients with acute herpes zoster. .* **Haanpaa M, Dastidar P, Weinberg A, et al.** 1998, Neurology 51(5):, pp. 1405-11.

30. Post-herpetic neuralgia - Treatment. *NHS choices.* [Online] 2014. [Cited: 3 26, 2017.] http://www.nhs.uk/Conditions/postherpetic-neuralgia/Pages/Treatment.aspx.

31. *Topical Capsaicin for Pain Management.* **Anand P, Bley K.** 2011, Br J Anaesth 107(4), pp. 490-502.

32. Capsaicin cream. *Drugs.com.* [Online] 3 1, 2017. [Cited: 3 8, 2017.] https://www.drugs.com/cdi/capsaicin-cream.html.

33. *Review of lidocaine patch 5% studies in the treatment of postherpetic neuralgia.* **Davies PS, Galer BS.** 2004, Drugs 64(9), pp. 937-47.

34. Lidocaine Patch. *Drugs.com.* [Online] [Cited: 3 8, 2017.] https://www.drugs.com/cdi/lidocaine-patch.html.

35. EMLA. *Drugs.com.* [Online] [Cited: 3 26, 2017.] https://www.drugs.com/sfx/emla-side-effects.html.

36. *Chronic opioid therapy as alternative treatment for post-herpetic neuralgia.* **Pappagallo M, Campbell JN.** 1994, Ann Neurol. 35, pp. 54-6.

37. **Panickar A, Serpell M.** Guidelines for General Practitioners on Treatment of Pain in Post-Herpetic Neuralgia . [Online] 2015. [Cited: 3 12, 2017.] https://herpes.org.uk/wp-content/uploads/2015/10/Guidelines-for-PHN-by-Dr-Serpell.pdf.

38. *Continuous subcutaneous administration of the N-methyl-D-aspartic acid (NMDA) receptor antagonist ketamine in the treatment of post-herpetic neuralgia.* **Eide K, Stubhaug A, Oye I, Breivik H.** 1995, Pain 61(2), pp. 221-8.

39. *Topical amitriptyline and ketamine for post-herpetic neuralgia and other forms of neuropathic pain.* **Sawynok J, Zinger C.** 2016, Expert Opin Pharmacother.17(4), pp. 601-9.

40. *Treatment of Neuropathic Pain.* **K., Jefferies.** 2010, Semin Neurol 30(4), pp. 425-32 .

41. Antidepressants: Another weapon against chronic pain. *Mayo Clinic.* [Online] 2016. [Cited: 3 20, 2017.] http://www.mayoclinic.org/pain-medications/art-20045647?pg=2.

42. Treatment of Neuropathic Pain. *MedScape.* [Online] 2010. [Cited: 3 20, 2017.] http://www.medscape.com/viewarticle/730671_3.

43. *Acute Administration of Gabapentin Can Prevent Postherpetic Neuralgia.* **F., Lowry.** 2011, American Academy of Dermatology.

44. *Treatment of postherpetic neuralgia: focus on pregabalin.* **KA., Cappuzzo.** 2009, Clin Interv Aging 4, pp. 17–23.

45. **P., Dreyfuss.** Sympathetic Nerve Block Information. *spine universe.* [Online] 2016. [Cited: 3 27, 2017.] https://www.spineuniverse.com/treatments/pain-management/sympathetic-nerve-block-information.

46. *Caudal Epidural of Pulsed Radiofrequency in Post Herpetic Neuralgia (PHN); Report of Three Cases.* **OJJM., Rohof.** 2014, Anesthesiology and Pain Medicine 4(3), pp. 163-9.

47. *Thoracoscopic sympathectomy: techniques and outcomes.* **al., Johnson JP et.** 1998, Neurosurg Focus 4 (2).

48. Continuous Thoracic Paravertebral Block. *NYSORA-Nw+ew York school of regional anaesthesia.* [Online] 2013. [Cited: 4 4, 2017.] http://www.nysora.com/techniques/neuraxial-and-perineuraxial-techniques/landmark-based/3033-continuous-thoracic-paravertebral-block.html.

49. *Intrathecal steroid therapy for postherpetic neuralgia: a review.* **Nelson DA, Landau WM.** 2002, Expert Rev Neurother 2(5), pp. 631-7.

50. *Response of Intractable Post Herpetic Neuralgia to Intrathecal Baclofen.* **Hosny A, Simopoulos T, Collins B.** 2004, Pain Physician 7, pp. 345-7.

51. *Intrathecal Medications in Post-Herpetic Neuralgia.* **Fabiano Aj, Doyle C, Plunkett RJ.** 2012, Pain Med 13(8): , pp. 1088–90.

52. *History of the development of corticosteroid therapy.* **TG., Benedek.** 2011, Clin Exp Rheumatol 29(68), pp. 5-12.

53. *Herpes Zoster and Postherpetic Neuralgia: Prevention and Management.* **Mounsey AL, Matthew LG, Slawson DC.** 2005, Am Fam Physician. 15;72(6), pp. 1075-80.

54. *Physical exercise as non-pharmacological treatment of chronic pain: Why and when. .* **Ambrose KR, Golightly YM.** 2015, Best practice & research Clinical rheumatology. 29(1), pp. 120-130.

55. *Transcutaneous electrical nerve stimulation for chronic post-herpetic neuralgia.* **Ing MR, Hellreich PD, Johnson DW, Chen JJ.** 2015, Int J Dermatol. 54(4), pp. 476-80.

56. *Transcutaneous electrical nerve stimulation (TENS).Mechanisms, Clinical Application and Evidence.* **M., Johnson.** 2007, Reviews in Pain. 1(1), pp. 7-11.

57. **team, Pain and symptom control.** *Percutaneous Electrical Nerve Stimulation (PENS).* Manchester : The Christie NHS Foundation Trust, 2014.

58. *An outpatient program in behavioral medicine for chronic pain patients based on the practice of mindfulness meditation: theoretical considerations and preliminary results.* **J, Kabat-Zinn.** 1982, Gen Hosp Psychiatry.4(1), pp. 33-47.

59. *Mindfulness meditation in older adults with postherpetic neuralgia: a randomized controlled pilot study.* **Meize-Grochowski R, Shuster G, Boursaw B, et al.** 2015, Geriatric nursing (New York, NY) 36(2), pp. 154-60.

60. Vitamins and supplements. *Web MD*. [Online] 2009. [Cited: 4 9, 2017.]

61. **SH, Hochschuler.** How to Use Ice Massage Therapy for Back Pain. *Spine-health*. [Online] 2006. [Cited: 4 9, 2017.] http://www.spine-health.com/treatment/heat-therapy-cold-therapy/how-use-ice-massage-therapy-back-pain.

62. *Effects of ice massage on neuropathic pain in persons with AIDS.* **KK., Ownby.** 2006, J Assoc Nurses AIDS Care 17(5), pp. 15-22.

63. *Management of Herpes Zoster (Shingles) and Postherpetic Neuralgia.* **Stankus SJ, Dlugopolski M, Packer D.** 2000, Am Fam Physician 15;61(8), pp. 2437-44.

64. *Herpes Zoster (Shingles) and Postherpetic Neuralgia.* . **Sampathkumar P, Drage LA, Martin DP.** 2009, Mayo Clinic Proceedings 84(3), pp. 274-80.

65. **Macres SM, Richeimer SH, Duran PJ.** Understanding neuropathic pain. *Help for pain*. [Online] 2000. [Cited: 3 2, 2017.] http://www.helpforpain.com/articles/understand-neuropathic-pain/understanding.htm.

Contents

Introduction 2

Chapter 1 3

Etiology 3

   Herpes zoster (Shingles) virus and varicella 3

   Herpes zoster or shingles 5

   Epidemiology 5

Chapter 2 Symptoms of shingles 10

Types and localisation of the herpes zoster 11

   Trigeminal shingles (herpes zoster) 11

      Ophthalmic region 13

      Maxillary region 15

      Mandibular region 16

      Auriculotemporal region 17

   Facial herpes zoster and Ramsay Hunt syndrome 18

   Herpes zoster of the skin of torso (dorsal spinal ganglions) ... 20

   Other areas of shingles less common 23

   Zoster sine herpete or Shingles without rash 26

   Complications of shingles and their treatment 27

   Neurological disorders of herpes zoster 30

Chapter 3 Neuralgia and postherpetic neuralgia 33

   Postherpetic neuralgia 34

   Pathophysiology and theories of development 34

   Symptoms 37

    Epidemiology of postherpetic neuralgia. How many people with shingles will develop this type of pain and when? 44

Chapter 4 Diagnosis 48
    Differential diagnosis 51

Chapter 5 Treatment 53
    First care for pain 53
        Cold compresses 53
        Capsaicin creams and skin patch 53
        Lidocaine skin patch and lidocaine cream (Lidoderm) 55
        EMLA cream 56
    Analgesics 56
        NSAID 57
        Opioid analgesics 57
        Ketamine and N-methyl-D-aspartate (NMDA) Receptor Antagonists 59
    Antidepressants 60
    Anticonvulsives 64
    Sympathetic nerve blocks 66
    Injection of the local anesthetics 68
    Radiofrequency ablation and pulsed radiofrequency lesioning 69
    Surgical procedures : 72
    Endoscopic (surgical) and chemical sympathectomy 72
    Injections in the deep tissue 75
    Injections to the spine-epidural injections 75
    Paravertebral injections 76

Intrathecal medication-direct effects on the brain surface 77
Steroid injections.. 79
Spinal cord stimulation (neurostimulation)............................. 81
Physical treatment 82
Percutaneous electrical nerve stimulation/transcutaneous electrical nerve stimulation 84
Adjunctive treatment... 88
Prognosis after treatment 94
Chapter 6 Prevention.. 96
Preventive measures.. 96
Treatment of herpes zoster 96
Vaccination 99
Works Cited 101

CPSIA information can be obtained
at www.ICGtesting.com
Printed in the USA
BVOW09s1726201017
498238BV00018B/279/P